About IFPRI and the 2020 Vision Initiative

The International Food Policy Research Institute (IFPRI) was established in 1975 as one of 15 centers supported by the Consultative Group on International Agricultural Research (CGIAR), an alliance of governments, private foundations, and international and regional organizations engaged in research for sustainable development. To contribute to a world free of poverty, hunger, and malnutrition, IFPRI conducts research on a wide range of topics, including agricultural productivity, global trade and local markets, maternal and early childhood nutrition, climate change, and individual country development strategies, among others. Based in Washington, DC, IFPRI has 12 offices worldwide including regional offices in Ethiopia, India, and Senegal.

The 2020 Vision for Food, Agriculture, and the Environment is an IFPRI initiative to develop a shared vision and consensus for action for meeting future world food needs while reducing poverty and protecting the environment. Through the 2020 Vision Initiative, IFPRI brings together divergent schools of thought on these issues, generates research, and develops policy recommendations.

IFPRI's research, capacity-strengthening, and communications activities are made possible by its financial contributors and partners. IFPRI receives its principal funding from governments, private foundations, and international and regional organizations, most of which are members of the CGIAR. IFPRI gratefully acknowledges the generous unrestricted funding from Australia, Canada, China, Denmark, Finland, France, Germany, India, Ireland, the Netherlands, Norway, South Africa, Sweden, Switzerland, the United Kingdom, the United States, and the World Bank.

D0293381

Reshaping Agriculture for Nutrition and Health

Reshaping Agriculture for Nutrition and Health

An IFPRI 2020 Book

Edited by Shenggen Fan and Rajul Pandya-Lorch

International Food Policy Research Institute
Washington, DC

International Food Policy Research Institute
2033 K Street, NW
Washington, DC 20006-1002, USA
Telephone: +1-202-862-5600
www.ifpri.org

DOI: 10.2499/9780896296732

Library of Congress Cataloging-in-Publication Data

Reshaping agriculture for nutrition and health / edited by Shenggen Fan and
    Rajul Pandya-Lorch.
        p. cm.
    Includes bibliographical references.
    ISBN 978-0-89629-673-2 (alk. paper)
    1. Food supply. 2. Nutrition policy. 3. Agriculture. 4. Public health.
I. Fan, Shenggen. II. Pandya-Lorch, Rajul. III. International Food Policy
Research Institute.
HD9000.6.R47 2012
363.8'7—dc23

                                                                    2012001948

Cover design: Julia Vivalo / Book layout: David Popham.

Contents

Preface

Persistent hunger, malnutrition, and ill health threaten the ability of many countries to achieve the Millennium Development Goals by 2015. What happens in the agriculture sector—a supplier of food and essential nutrients, a source of income and employment, and an engine of growth—has important implications for nutrition and health. With the recent food crises, agriculture, for the first time in two decades, is high on the global agenda. The International Food Policy Research Institute (IFPRI) and its 2020 Vision Initiative decided to leverage this momentum to inform, influence, and catalyze key actors to better use agricultural investments to sustainably reduce malnutrition and improve health for the world's most vulnerable people.

This book is intended to identify knowledge gaps, foster new thinking, and stimulate concrete actions on leveraging agriculture for improving nutrition and health. It is meant to serve a variety of audiences, from scholars, academics, students, and researchers, to practitioners working on the ground, to decisionmakers devising policies that successfully connect agriculture, nutrition, and health at the local, regional, and global levels. Readers interested in probing these topics more fully can follow the references to the discussion papers, journal articles, and books that underlie many of the chapters.

This book is a compilation of peer-reviewed background papers and briefs commissioned by IFPRI for the international conference "Leveraging Agriculture for Improving Nutrition and Health," which took place in New Delhi in February 2011. We hope this book will inspire dialogue within and between sectors, as a first step toward shaping agricultural investments that improve human nutrition and health around the world.

Shenggen Fan
Director General, IFPRI

Rajul Pandya-Lorch
Head, 2020 Vision Initiative, IFPRI

Acknowledgments

The chapters in this book were originally commissioned as background papers and briefs for "Leveraging Agriculture for Improving Nutrition and Health," a global conference facilitated by the IFPRI 2020 Vision Initiative and hosted in New Delhi in February 2011. Authors include IFPRI senior staff and other leading researchers, practitioners, and policymakers from around the world. All of the conference papers and briefs were peer reviewed (or based on peer-reviewed materials) before they were made available to conference participants. Subsequently, in preparation for this book, all of the briefs were converted into book chapters and underwent further peer review by IFPRI's independent Publications Review Committee. We thank the Committee and its chair, Gershon Feder, for these careful and timely reviews.

We are deeply grateful to the policy consultations and conference process cosponsors that made this book possible: Asian Development Bank, Bill & Melinda Gates Foundation, Canadian International Development Agency, Technical Centre for Agricultural and Rural Cooperation (CTA), Deutsche Gesellschaft für Internationale Zusammenarbeit (GIZ) GmbH, International Fund for Agricultural Development (IFAD), Indian Economic Association, International Development Research Centre, Canada/Le Centre de recherches pour le développement international, Irish Aid, PepsiCo, UK Department for International Development (DFID), United States Agency for International Development (USAID) and its Feed the Future Initiative, and the World Bank. We also gratefully acknowledge IFPRI's unrestricted funding from Australia, Canada, China, Denmark, Finland, France, Germany, India, Ireland, the Netherlands, Norway, South Africa, Sweden, Switzerland, the United Kingdom, the United States, and the World Bank, which enabled IFPRI to establish the 2020 Vision Initiative and the research base for the overarching work reported here.

We express our sincere appreciation to the authors of the chapters for their invaluable contributions that have enriched our knowledge base and enabled more informed discourse on how to make agriculture more nutrition and health friendly.

We warmly thank our colleagues for their tremendous support throughout the preparation of this book and its underlying background papers and briefs: Evelyn Banda, Adrienne Chu, Djhoanna Cruz, Kenda Cunningham, Heidi Fritschel, Corinne Garber, Michael Go, Zhenya Karelina, Vickie Lee, David Popham, Gwendolyn Stansbury, Ashley St. Thomas, Julia Vivalo, Klaus von Grebmer, John Whitehead, and Sivan Yosef.

Chapter 1

Overview

Shenggen Fan, Rajul Pandya-Lorch, and Heidi Fritschel

Most people would say agriculture is about growing food; they are right. Agricultural performance, after all, is measured in terms of production—for example, yield or grain production. The purpose of agriculture, however, does not stop there. At a deeper level, the purpose of agriculture is not just to grow crops and livestock for food and raw materials, but to grow healthy, well-nourished people. One of farmers' most important tasks is to produce food of sufficient quantity (that is, enough calories) and quality (with the vitamins and minerals needed by the human body) to feed all of the planet's people sustainably so they can lead healthy, productive lives. This is effectively one of the goals of agriculture, although it is rarely made explicit.

Could agriculture do more to meet this goal? Recently the international development community has turned its attention to the potential for the agriculture, nutrition, and health sectors to work together to enhance human well-being. In some ways, of course, agriculture, health, and nutrition are already deeply entwined. Agricultural production is an important means for most people to get the food and essential nutrients they need. And in many poor countries, where agriculture is highly labor intensive, productive agriculture requires the labor of healthy, well-nourished people. Yet, in other ways agriculture, health, and nutrition are quite separate: professionals in these three fields usually work in isolation from one another, with their efforts sometimes dovetailing in mutually beneficial ways and sometimes working at cross-purposes.

In an ideal world, consumers would be fully aware of the merits of nutritious foods, and producers, processors, and marketers, in turn, would know how to produce, process, and market these high-quality, nutrient-rich foods. Market forces would provide the incentives, through product prices, to all involved in producing or consuming nutrient-rich foods. Unfortunately, our world is less than ideal, and market prices do not provide an adequate incentive for producing nutritious food. And, even if prices did reflect the nutritional value of food, they could put nutritious foods out of reach of poor people. This means public interventions are needed to correct market failures (when prices do not reflect the nutritional value of foods) or to improve affordability (for poor people).

How much more could agriculture do to improve human well-being if it included specific actions and interventions to achieve health and nutrition goals? What kinds of changes would maximize agriculture's contribution to human health and nutrition, and how could human health and nutrition contribute to a productive and sustainable agricultural system?

Room for Improvement

Over the past century or so, agricultural development has been based on a paradigm of increasing productivity and maximizing the production of cereals. This paradigm has produced an agricultural system that is the world's primary source of calories and employs 60–80 percent of people in low-income countries (IFC 2009). The ramping up of cereal production in the Green Revolution, for example, saved countless lives in Asia (Hazell 2009), and agricultural growth there has served as a springboard for a blistering pace of economic growth, improving the lives of millions. At the same time, agricultural intensification has led to a concentration on grain production; crowded out nutrient-dense crops like pulses, fruits, and vegetables; increased the risk of agriculture-associated diseases; led to the development of new diseases (such as the evolving forms of influenza); and exacerbated environmental degradation that can have negative consequences for human health. Moreover, millions of smallholders who produce food still suffer from poverty and hunger, and recent food price hikes have made those who are net buyers of food even more vulnerable.

A look at the current global health and nutrition situation suggests agriculture can make an even greater contribution to health and nutrition. Indeed, leveraging agriculture for health and nutrition has the potential to speed progress toward meeting all eight of the Millennium Development Goals. The world's farmers already provide billions of people with diverse, healthy diets—yet more needs to be done. About one-seventh of the world's population is going hungry (FAO and WFP 2010). In developing countries, one out of four children—about 146 million in all—is underweight (UNICEF 2006). Millions of people suffer from serious vitamin and mineral deficiencies. For example, vitamin A deficiency compromises the immune systems of about 40 percent of children younger than age five in developing countries and results in the early deaths of about 1 million young children each year. Iron deficiency impairs the mental development of 40–60 percent of the developing world's children aged 6 to 24 months and leads to the deaths of about 50,000 women a year during pregnancy and childbirth (Micronutrient Initiative and UNICEF 2004). The economic cost of micronutrient deficiencies is estimated to be 2.4–10.0 percent of gross domestic product (GDP) in many developing countries (Stein and Qaim 2007). Thus the Copenhagen Consensus has ranked vitamin

A and zinc supplements for children and iron and iodine fortification of food as numbers one and three, respectively, in its solutions to the most important human challenges (Copenhagen Consensus Center 2008). Hunger and malnutrition have effects that last throughout the life cycle, with poorly nourished children growing up to be less healthy and productive than they could be. Girls who do not get the nutrition they need are at great risk of becoming undernourished women who, in turn, are at increased risk of giving birth to the next generation of undernourished children (ACC/SCN 2000).

While some people are getting too little food, others are getting too much of the wrong food. Diets centered on cheap, calorie-dense, nutrient-poor foods (including both "fast foods" and nutrient-poor staples) are deepening the emerging epidemic of obesity and chronic diseases in countries undergoing economic and nutrition transitions. Overweight affects more than 1 billion people globally, and obesity affects at least 300 million. Since 1980, obesity rates have risen threefold or more in some areas of North America, the United Kingdom, Eastern Europe, the Middle East, the Pacific Islands, Australasia, and China (WHO 2010; Nugent 2011).

The chapters in this volume look at the links among agriculture, nutrition, and health and their potential to convey more benefits to poor and hungry people. The authors come at the issues from many perspectives, examining not only the overall links among the three sectors, but also the specific roles played by economic and agricultural growth, innovations in crop science and food supply chains, the health of agricultural laborers, agriculture-associated diseases, women's place at the intersection of the three sectors, and the challenges of advocacy and policymaking.

Conceptualizing the Links

In Chapter 2 of this volume, John Hoddinott describes a conceptual framework that clarifies the links among agriculture, nutrition, and health. This framework includes the physical, social, legal, governance, and economic settings in which people live and work; the resources—time and capital—at their disposal; and the processes associated with agricultural production and determinants of health and nutritional status. These elements of the framework suggest pathways through which agricultural production and markets can affect health and nutrition, including changes in incomes, crop varieties, production methods, and allocation of resources within households. A clear framework that shows the relationships among agriculture, nutrition, and health can help decisionmakers exploit the links in policies and programs.

It is also possible to look beyond agriculture to the whole food system and its interaction with nutrition and health (see Chapter 3 by Per Pinstrup-Andersen). The food system includes not only agriculture but also natural resources and inputs;

transport, storage, and exchange; secondary production; and consumption. Each of these food system activities can interact with health and nutrition, in both obvious and less obvious ways. Integrated actions related to, for example, zoonotic diseases, HIV/AIDS, crop protection, sustainable management of natural resources, and food safety can not only promote agricultural productivity, but also improve nutrition and health and help overcome poverty traps.

The Role of Growth in Improving Nutrition

It is natural to assume that economic growth has a positive impact on people's nutritional status through increased incomes and food expenditures, but the limited evidence available shows that, in a number of developing countries, economic growth has failed to result in better nutrition.

Various studies show that in many agrarian countries agricultural growth is more effective than growth in other sectors in reducing undernutrition (see Chapter 4 by Shenggen Fan and Joanna Brzeska and Chapter 5 by Derek Headey). The composition of growth, the distribution of growth, and the conditions under which growth takes place all matter. Growth in agricultural subsectors where poor people are engaged, such as staple crops, contributes more to reducing poverty and increasing calorie intake than growth in, for instance, export crops. Later in the development process, growth in other sectors besides agriculture becomes more important in improving food and nutrition security. Neither agricultural nor nonagricultural growth alone, however, is sufficient to reduce child undernutrition or micronutrient malnutrition (see Chapter 6 by Olivier Ecker, Clemens Breisinger, and Karl Pauw and Chapter 7 by Karl Pauw and James Thurlow). Complementary programs in nutrition, health, water and sanitation, and behavior change communication also need to be implemented and targeted to vulnerable populations, especially women and young children. More broadly, improvements in healthcare access and female education and reductions in fertility rates and poverty will help make nutrition more responsive to growth.

Despite great strides in food production, agricultural growth has not had its expected benefits for nutrition in India, which is home to one-third of the world's undernourished children (see Chapter 20 by Stuart Gillespie and Suneetha Kadiyala). One part of the solution to this "Indian enigma" likely involves focusing on crops and livestock that have large nutritional impacts on both farmers and consumers. Another part may involve addressing socioeconomic factors that affect the link between agriculture and nutrition, including the distribution of assets, particularly land; the role and social status of women; rural infrastructure; and rural health and sanitation. Yet another part involves addressing other drivers of undernutrition by, for example, improving education and social welfare systems.

Opportunities to Meet the Challenge

Although the agriculture, health, and nutrition sectors all seek to improve human well-being, agriculture has rarely been explicitly deployed in this way. However, opportunities exist all along the agricultural value chain to improve nutrition and reduce health risks. In Chapter 9, Corinna Hawkes and Marie T. Ruel examine how a value-chain approach to development can incorporate nutrition goals and thereby make nutritious foods more available and affordable for the poor. This approach starts by looking at every component of the food supply chain from the field to the table—including production, postharvest processing, marketing, and trade—and determining where value for nutrition can be integrated. Incentives are created in ways that do not interfere with the creation of economic value for supply-chain actors. New initiatives are emerging in several developing countries to explore the value-chain approach's potential to improve nutrition.

Another innovation for leveraging agriculture to improve nutrition is biofortification—the breeding of new varieties of food crops with improved nutritional content. When people in malnourished communities receive these varieties to grow and eat, biofortified crops can contribute to the overall reduction of micronutrient deficiencies in a population. Compared with other approaches to micronutrient malnutrition, such as supplementation and fortification, biofortification offers several advantages: it targets poor people and rural areas; it is cost-effective because after the initial investment in research, the crops are available year after year; and it is sustainable because it relies on staple crops that people are already accustomed to eating. A pilot program in Mozambique and Uganda that has disseminated varieties of orange sweet potato with high levels of vitamin A has already shown increased vitamin A intakes in vulnerable groups (see Chapter 10 by Howarth Bouis and Yassir Islam). Successful results depend on high levels of bioavailability or bioconversion of the nutrients and high rates of farmer and consumer adoption.

Part of the pressure on the global food system in recent years has come from rising incomes and rapid urbanization in developing countries, which have increased global food demand. IFPRI's International Model for Policy Analysis of Agricultural Commodities and Trade (IMPACT) shows that rich countries' dietary shift toward healthier and less-meat-intensive diets could increase calorie availability and reduce child malnutrition in poor countries. This finding suggests governments in rich countries should consider encouraging consumers to move away from meat-intensive diets through, for example, nutrition education and government-sponsored feeding programs (see Chapter 8 by Siwa Msangi and Mark W. Rosegrant).

While agriculture can improve health through improved incomes or improved nutrition, it may also increase risks for certain diseases. Additionally, the food value chain involves many hazards: microbiological hazards, such as food-borne pathogens; physical and chemical hazards, such as plant toxins and pesticides; and occupational hazards, such as accidents. Poor people face challenges in producing and consuming safe food. Policymakers are increasingly using risk analysis to help them decide on regulatory and other actions to reduce health risks along the food value chain (see Chapter 11 by Pippa Chenevix Trench, Clare Narrod, Devesh Roy, and Marites Tiongco).

Another way of classifying agriculture-associated diseases is based on transmission pathways; high-burden categories include zoonoses, food-associated diseases, water-associated diseases, and occupational diseases. Such diseases sicken and kill billions of people a year and impose enormous economic costs, especially on poor countries. It is important to assess the full costs of these diseases, not only to human health but also to agricultural productivity, the food economy, and the ecosystem. Because the causes and effects of these diseases are complex, they call for interventions that integrate several sectors, including agriculture and livestock production, human medicine, veterinary medicine, and environmental science (see Chapter 12 by John McDermott and Delia Grace). Malaria, for example, is often linked to irrigation development and changes in land use associated with agriculture. It imposes heavy healthcare costs on small-farm households and impedes agricultural development by leading to declines in labor. The problem of malaria makes a clear case for coordination of health and agricultural policies (see Chapter 15 by Kwadwo Asenso-Okyere, Felix A. Asante, Jifar Tarekegn, and Kwaw S. Andam).

It is clear that disease cuts the productivity of farm labor in both the short and long terms and that farm labor itself can harm people's health and nutrition status. This means that health and agriculture interventions should be designed with these two-way linkages in mind. But does it follow that health investments necessarily improve agricultural productivity? Research on this question is sparse. The available evidence suggests that some inexpensive health interventions (such as micronutrient supplements) can have large effects, that health interventions are most effective when combined with education and infrastructure investments, and that improving children's health can lead to increased adult productivity in the long term (see Chapter 13 by Paul E. McNamara, John M. Ulimwengu, and Kenneth L. Leonard and Chapter 14 by Kwadwo Asenso-Okyere, Catherine Chiang, Paul Thangata, and Kwaw S. Andam).

Women are an important group linking agricultural development and human health and nutrition. They are not only responsible for food preparation and caring for young children and ill household members, but in many countries women are also the main agricultural producers. Strengthening women's position both within the agricultural sector and within the household can significantly improve households' nutrition and health. Experiences from several agricultural development strategies show much scope exists for increasing women's access to and control over resources, such as household income (see Chapter 16 by Ruth Meinzen-Dick, Julia Behrman, Purnima Menon, and Agnes Quisumbing).

Policymaking across Sectors

Making policies that leverage agriculture for nutrition and health poses particular challenges. Malnutrition and poor health are the result of many factors and require action in a whole range of sectors. Although the health and agriculture sectors have well-established institutions within government, they are not organized in ways that readily allow for cross-sectoral action. And the nutrition sector often lacks a high-profile place in government. It suffers from a lack of awareness about the consequences of and solutions to malnutrition, weak commitment from political leaders, and limited resources for public investment. Nonetheless, there are ways to promote action on nutrition and across sectors, including advocacy by civil society and community groups and the cultivation of policy champions (well-connected and well-informed people with access to the policy process). Agriculture-associated health problems require joint agriculture and health solutions. Achieving these joint solutions may involve creating incentives for intersectoral collaboration, implementing multisectoral policy reviews, carrying out health-impact studies of agricultural development projects, and promoting joint agriculture, nutrition, and health policy formulation and planning (see Chapter 17 by Todd Benson, Chapter 18 by Robert Mwadime, Chapter 19 by Brenda Shenute Namugumya, and Chapter 21 by Joachim von Braun, Marie T. Ruel, and Stuart Gillespie).

The best approach to finding positive synergies among agriculture, nutrition, and health may depend on a country's position in the dietary transition, where stage one is a diet low in calories and micronutrients, stage two is a diet adequate in calories for most people but with inadequate micronutrients, and stage three is a diet that provides excessive calories, still with possible micronutrient deficiencies. In stage one countries, government's primary task is to provide public goods that contribute to improvements in agriculture, nutrition, and health, such as infrastructure, education, and health services. During stage two, the task is to deliver targeted agricultural, nutritional, and health services to people who do not experience the benefits of growth. At stage three, governments must regulate the growing private sector, including commercial farms, food manufacturers, retailers, and restaurants (see Chapter 22 by Robert Paarlberg).

Breaking down the siloes between the sectors will require a change in thinking. Education in all three sectors can do more to highlight the synergies among them and develop a shared body of knowledge that will follow students into their professional lives. Professionals in the three sectors should retain their deep expertise in their subject areas, while also gaining a greater familiarity with the other sectors' main concerns and opportunities. By developing cross-disciplinary programs, educational institutions can produce graduates and professionals who—in their capacity as extension workers, healthcare providers, or nutrition counselors—can effectively translate the linkages among agriculture, health, and nutrition in the field for the benefit of all. In addition, evaluations of projects and programs in all three sectors should take the other sectors into account, to help implementers gain feedback and to create incentives for collaboration.

Regional Experiences

The links between the three sectors—and consequently, potential solutions—will undoubtedly look different in different countries and regions, given the variations in agricultural systems and practices, food systems, and health and nutrition status. Initial efforts in some countries can point the way to potentially effective approaches and show what works and what does not. It is important to examine how successes can be adapted and scaled up in different regions because the lessons learned from experience to date will suggest areas for investment and policy change.

In Africa, poor nutrition and health remain persistent problems. Although a new focus on agriculture in the region presents an opportunity for countries to exploit the links among agriculture, nutrition, and health as they revise their agricultural policies and direct more funding to the sector, many policymakers at the national, district, and local levels still do not see nutrition as a development issue that should play a role in agricultural planning—despite the existence of several programs linking the sectors in that region. Raising nutrition's profile in African policymaking circles will thus require strong advocacy from civil society to senior policymakers.

In South Asia, malnutrition is disturbingly high. Important questions remain about why strong economic growth in the region, especially in India, has not done more to push down rates of malnutrition there. It is clear, however, that investments are needed to improve safety net systems and targeted nutrition programs; increase the production and consumption of nutritious foods; enhance gender equity; and strengthen agricultural technologies, rural infrastructure, information technology, and irrigation, water, sanitation, agricultural extension, and credit systems. In addition, programs often rely on nongovernmental organizations (NGOs) for funding and support; when NGO funding stops, so do the programs. Consequently, it is important to ensure program sustainability to improve people's nutrition and health.

Although East Asia does not suffer from as much undernutrition as some other regions, problems of malnutrition remain. For a number of countries in East Asia, agriculture means rice production. Impressive gains in the productivity of rice farmers in recent decades have helped raise incomes and reduce hunger.

Nonetheless, many farmers still have problems getting access to high-quality seeds, fertilizers, water, rural infrastructure, and machinery for processing. It is also important to promote more diverse diets and educate farmers in the region about the potential for growing more nutritious crops, such as fruits and vegetables. A holistic, community-based approach to linking agriculture, nutrition, and health has worked well in some countries, including Thailand. Experience there shows the importance of teaching people about nutrition at the community level, teaching agricultural skills, and making sure farmers have the land, credit, and postharvest technologies they need.

Walking the line between undernutrition and overnutrition has proven difficult in many parts of the world. In Latin America, hunger overlaps with overweight and obesity, sometimes even in the same family, so efforts are needed to deal with both undernutrition and health problems related to overnutrition. Argentina, for example, has recognized that overweight is concentrated among its poor citizens. Joint public and private action is needed to help reduce sugar, salt, and saturated fat in manufactured food products. Brazil has one of the world's largest school feeding programs, which brings together agriculture, nutrition, and health, but poverty- and hunger-related social programs have not yet reached all poor and marginalized groups, so more remains to be done.

Finally, in the high-income countries, overweight and obesity are reaching epidemic levels. In many of these countries, government policies are designed to maximize the export value of crops and enable low food prices at home, with deleterious effects on the health and nutrition of citizens. Unfortunately, evidence of cost-effective countrywide approaches to decreasing overweight and obesity is extremely scant. As with micronutrient interventions, overweight and obesity prevention will likely need a much more multisectoral approach. Educational programs on nutrition and health in schools and communities can build awareness, but they must also take into account the psychology of consumers and the difficulty of changing their behaviors.

Looking Ahead

The world food system, where the agriculture, health, and nutrition sectors come together, faces serious challenges in the coming years. High and volatile food prices are likely to be a reality for the foreseeable future. They pose difficulties not only for food consumers, who often shift their diets to cheaper, less-nutritious foods, but also for food producers, who may reduce their investments in agriculture in the face of increased input prices and uncertain output prices. Rising populations and changing diets are putting pressure on farmers to produce more food with the same resources. And climate change creates risks for agriculture and health—and by extension, nutrition—that are only beginning to be understood. This is the context in which decisionmakers at all levels and in many sectors will need to act (see Chapter 23 by Shenggen Fan, Rajul Pandya-Lorch, and Heidi Fritschel).

At the same time, attention to the agricultural sector is growing, along with an interest in leveraging agriculture for nutrition and health. Now is an ideal time to look for solutions that will not only help make the agricultural system highly productive and sustainable, but also maximize its contributions to human well-being.

References

ACC/SCN (Administrative Committee on Coordination/Subcommittee on Nutrition). 2000. *Fourth Report on the World Nutrition Situation.* Geneva: ACC/SCN in collaboration with the International Food Policy Research Institute.

Bryce, J., C. Boschi-Pinto, K. Shibuya, R. E. Black, and the WHO Child Health Epidemiology Group. 2005. "WHO Estimates of the Causes of Death in Children." *The Lancet* 365: 1147–1152.

Copenhagen Consensus Center. 2008. *Copenhagen Consensus 2008.* www.copenhagenconsensus. com/Home.aspx.

Diao, X., P. Hazell, D. Resnick, and J. Thurlow. 2007. *The Role of Agriculture in Development: Implications for Sub-Saharan Africa.* Research Report 153. Washington, DC: International Food Policy Research Institute.

FAO and ILO (Food and Agriculture Organization of the United Nations and International Labor Organization). n.d. FAQs: Some Selected Issues. Pathways out of Poverty. www.fao-ilo.org/ fileadmin/user_upload/fao_ilo/pdf/FAQs/Main_issues__2_.pdf.

FAO and WFP (Food and Agriculture Organization of the United Nations and World Food Programme). 2010. *The State of Food Insecurity in the World: Addressing Food Insecurity in Protracted Crises.* Rome.

Hazell, P. B. R. 2009. "Transforming Agriculture: The Green Revolution in Asia." In *Millions Fed: Proven Successes in Agricultural Development,* edited by David J. Spielman and Rajul Pandya-Lorch. Washington, DC: International Food Policy Research Institute.

IFC (International Finance Corporation). 2009. *IFC and Agribusiness.* IFC Issue Brief. Washington, DC.

Micronutrient Initiative and UNICEF (United Nations Children's Fund). 2004. *Vitamin and Mineral Deficiency: A Global Damage Assessment Report.* Ottawa, Canada, and New York. www.micronutrient.org/CMFiles/PubLib/Report-67-VMD-A-Global-Damage-Assessment-Report1KSB-3242008-9634.pdf.

Nugent, R. 2011. *Bringing Agriculture to the Table: How Agriculture and Food Can Play a Role in Preventing Chronic Disease.* Chicago: Chicago Council on Global Affairs.

Stein, A., and M. Qaim. 2007. "The Human and Economic Cost of Hidden Hunger." *Food and Nutrition Bulletin* 28 (2): 125–134.

UNICEF (United Nations Children's Fund). 2006. *The State of the World's Children 2007.* New York.

WFP (World Food Programme). 2010. "Hunger Stats." www.wfp.org/hunger/stats.

WHO (World Health Organization). 2010. Global Strategy on Diet, Physical Activity, and Health: Obesity and Overweight. www.who.int/dietphysicalactivity/publications/facts/obesity/en/index.html.

World Bank. 2007. "World Bank Calls for Renewed Emphasis on Agriculture for Development." Press release, October 19. http://web.worldbank.org/WBSITE/EXTERNAL/NEWS/0,,contentMDK:21517663~pagePK:64257043~piPK:437376~theSitePK:4607,00.html.

Chapter 2

Agriculture, Health, and Nutrition: Toward Conceptualizing the Linkages

John Hoddinott

Agriculture and health and nutrition have long occupied separate realms. Analyses of agricultural production seldom recognize that health status affects productivity, nor do they recognize that agricultural goods and processes have health consequences. At the policy and programmatic levels, agriculture and health operate in separate silos, seldom considering the consequences of their actions on sectors outside their own. This separation is strange given that agriculture and health and nutrition are tightly wedded. Agriculture is the primary source of calories and essential nutrients and is a major source of income for the world's poor, while agriculture-related health losses are massive.

Strengthening the policy and programmatic links between agriculture and health and nutrition requires a means of seeing how their myriad links fit together. This chapter sketches a framework that elucidates the channels through which agriculture affects health and nutrition and vice versa. While this framework can be applied at the global or national level, here it is focused on households and individuals, given that improving individual welfare is the ultimate goal of public policy.

The Basic Framework

The framework has three components: settings, resources, and the processes associated with agricultural production and the determinants of health and nutrition status.

Settings

The physical, social, legal, governance, and economic settings in which individuals live and work influence their actions. The *physical setting* refers to phenomena that affect agricultural production, such as the level and variability of rainfall, soil

This chapter is based on the author's 2020 Conference Paper, *Agriculture, Health, and Nutrition: Toward Conceptualizing the Linkages* (Washington, DC: International Food Policy Research Institute, 2011).

fertility, distances to markets, and quality of infrastructure. The physical environment also incorporates phenomena that directly affect human health—access to safe water and the presence of communicable human and zoonotic diseases being primary examples. The *social setting* captures such factors as the existence of trust, reciprocity, social cohesion, and strife. Norms of gender roles, "correct" behaviors, and folk wisdom—for example, what type of foods mothers "should" feed their children—are also part of the social setting.

The *legal setting* can be thought of as the rules that govern economic exchange. It affects agriculture through the restrictions it imposes on and the opportunities it creates for the production and sale of different foods, and through the regulation of labor and capital markets. The legal setting also affects health in terms of regulations applicable to the health sector in addition to those that govern food processing and safety. The *governance setting* captures how rules are developed, implemented, and enforced. It includes the political processes that create rules—for example, centralized or decentralized decisionmaking, dictatorial or democratic governance, and so on—and the implementation of these rules through bureaucracies, parastatals, and third-party organizations. Finally, the *economic setting* captures policies that affect the level, returns, and variability of returns on assets and, as such, influence choices regarding productive activities undertaken by individuals, firms, and households.

Resources

Households have resources—time and capital. Time refers to the availability of physical labor for work. Capital includes such assets as land, tools, livestock, social capital, financial resources, and human capital in the form of schooling and knowledge. It also includes human capital in the form of health and nutrition status. Some resources, such as health and schooling, are always held by individuals, while others, such as land, may be individually or collectively owned. These resources are allocated to different productive activities, including food production, cash-crop production, livestock raising, and nonagricultural income-generating activities, such as wage labor, handicrafts, and services.

Households may receive transfer income from other households or from the state. For smallholder households, agricultural production will be the predominant use of household resources. For landless or near-landless households, urban households, or households located in more advanced economies, wage labor or nonagricultural business activities will matter most. While differences in livelihoods do not change the basics of the framework presented in this brief, they imply that certain links among agriculture, health, and nutrition will be more important for some households than for others.

Agricultural Production

Agricultural production is affected by the settings within which the household resides, with the physical and economic settings being especially important. Both the natural physical setting—rainfall, temperature, soil quality, elevation, and so forth—and the man-made physical setting—roads, bridges, and other forms of infrastructure—influence what livestock can be raised, what crops can be grown and when, and the places where these products can be marketed. The economic setting—particularly the markets encountered by farmers—provides signals as to what activities are profitable and the types of inputs that can be profitably employed.

Within these settings, the household allocates its resources, capital, knowledge, and time. In some cases, allocations of all resources may be a collective decision. In other cases, individual men and women within the household may choose how to allocate the resources under their own control, independent of what other household members choose to do. In still other cases, some activities will be undertaken collectively or perhaps under the direction of one household member, while others are done individually.

In making these allocations, household members are also making choices about the technologies used in the generation of income. These technologies govern what crops will be produced, what livestock will be raised, how they will be produced, and when production will take place. Note that the health and nutrition status of individual members will affect the choice of activities, the timing of these activities, and the intensity with which productive activities will be undertaken. For example, individuals who are suffering from iron deficiencies or have a physical disability will encounter greater difficulty in using their physical labor to produce agricultural output. In populations where there are severe deficiencies in energy intake, or where economic activities are physically demanding, increased nutrient intake can raise labor productivity.

Savings and Consumption

Income can be saved or consumed. Savings create a feedback loop within this framework. Consumption decisions, in terms of the quantity and quality of goods consumed and the timing of this consumption, are affected by prices faced by households which in turn are a reflection of the structure, conduct, and performance of the markets with which households interact. Markets provide goods, such as medicine and clothing, that positively affect health status, as well as those that negatively affect health, such as tobacco. Food consumption—with its quantity, quality, and diversity dimensions—will account for a considerable fraction of the budgets of poor households.

Determinants of Health Status

The setting within which households and individuals live affects health. The physical setting—climate, access to water, the prevalence of communicable diseases, and health infrastructure—plays a major role in health status. So too does the social setting. Norms regarding what constitutes good health, the circumstances under which individuals should seek healthcare from modern or traditional sources, and how illnesses should be treated will all affect health status. Health is also affected by the allocation of individual and household resources. Assets in the form of the quality of housing and physical goods associated with water, sewerage, and waste disposal will affect health status. Knowledge of how health should be maintained, how illnesses can be identified, and how those illnesses can be treated will affect health. The allocation of time plays an important role in maintaining or improving health. Health status is also affected by the consumption of goods that directly improve or worsen health. Nutritional status affects health—for example, severe vitamin-A deficiencies lead to blindness.

The links between health status and agriculture are bidirectional. Choices made in agricultural production affect health through three channels. First, manual work in agriculture is physically demanding and can directly damage health. Second, agricultural work exposes individuals to harmful pathogens, such as those found in water-borne diseases or those that come from zoonotic sources. Third, where agricultural production involves the use of chemical pesticides, exposure to these can be another threat to health.

Determinants of Nutritional Status

Nutritional status results from the combination of time, physical assets, and knowledge of good nutritional practices, together with health status and the consumption of food. Food consumption, in terms of quantity, quality, and diversity, plays a major role in determining nutritional status and, as such, provides the most direct link between agriculture and nutrition. But it is not the only factor. There are physical assets involved such as cooking pots and utensils. The nutritional status of very young children will be affected by the frequency of feeding—this is an example of how allocation of time (here, time devoted to childcare) affects individuals' nutritional status. Social norms regarding foods and who "should" consume them, and knowledge of what are the right foods to consume and in what quantities also affect nutritional status. Because nutritional status depends on the capacity of the body to absorb nutrients, it is affected by other dimensions of an individual's health status, such as the presence of healthy intestinal mucosa. Finally, the nutritional status of an individual within a household depends on how the amount of food and other inputs into nutrition are allocated across members.

Leveraging Change to Agriculture to Affect Health and Nutrition

There are numerous locations within the framework where leverage can be applied to bring about changes. Levers are available to policymakers and other stakeholders, but they can also be operated by natural, market, or other forces.

Levers affecting agricultural production, emanating from either the public or private sector, operate at the level of settings, resources, production, and markets. For example, environmental programs that focus on soil and water conservation are levers that affect the physical setting. Infrastructure improvement affects both the level and type of agricultural production. Changes in the economic setting such as changes in exchange rates, tariffs, and openness to trade—which partly reflect globalization—will affect access to inputs and to new markets. Private and public actors can change value chains in ways that affect incomes received by farmers, the types of foods available to consumers, and prices faced by both producers and consumers.

Levers affecting agricultural production and markets will affect health and nutrition through six pathways.

1. *Changes to incomes:* When changes in agricultural production lead to increases in household income, the income can be used to purchase goods that affect health status. Better clothing and the ability of households to purchase improved healthcare are examples of this potential to improve health status, while the purchase of tobacco products will damage health. Higher incomes can be used to purchase more food, higher-quality food, and a more diverse diet. These will directly improve nutritional status. Higher incomes will affect health indirectly through their impact on nutritional status and directly where the food purchased has fewer pathogens and thereby reduces exposure to food- and water-borne diseases.

2. *Changes in crops, farm practices, and markets:* Changes in agricultural production can result in the introduction of new foods into diets. At the farm level, the introduction of new crops as a result of innovations in crop breeding (for example, biofortified foods) has the potential to improve both health and nutrition. At the level of local, regional, or national food markets, actions by the private sector, governments, or other actors can make existing foods produced within a country available to new markets. Reforming tariffs and reducing barriers to agricultural trade will permit the entry of foods only produced outside the country. Finally, changes in processing can also affect foods consumed. This can be beneficial, for example, where foods are fortified with micronutrients, or harmful, as in cases where processing introduces excessive levels of sodium.

3. *Changes to crop varieties and production methods:* Changes in the types of crops that are grown or changes in production processes may make agricultural work either more or less physically intensive. For example, mechanization will reduce the physical demands of agricultural labor, whereas crops that require greater manual weeding will increase it. They will also change exposure to pesticides, zoonoses, and work-related accidents.

4. *Changes to the use of time:* Where changes increase the returns to time spent in agriculture, households may increase the amount of labor they devote to agricultural production. If this labor does not come from outside the household and if it does not come from reduced leisure, then some other household activity will be affected. Households might reduce time spent on other income-generating activities, make greater use of child labor, or reduce time spent on the production of health or nutrition.

5. *Changes to savings:* Where changes in agricultural production result in higher incomes, individuals and households may choose to save some of these higher incomes in the form of assets that improve health.

6. *Changes in intrahousehold resource allocation:* Changes in agricultural production may result in changes in the allocation of resources within the household. If this change results in women earning greater income, it may affect how households spend money, how food is allocated, and what types of assets are accumulated.

It is not always clear whether a change in agricultural production will improve or worsen health and nutrition. Several factors are at play. *First, how large are the income effects of this change?* Are these gross or net (accounting for input costs) income changes? How does income derived from other, nonagricultural income sources change? How strong are the links between income changes and the dimension of health being considered, as mediated through changes in consumption of goods that affect health status? Does higher income cause households to purchase more food or foods of improved quality? Do households spend these higher incomes on goods that have no effect, or even a negative effect, on health and nutrition?

Second, how do these changes affect pathways through which agricultural production affects health directly? Are household members more exposed to zoonoses or to poisons such as those found in pesticides? Is more time spent in agriculture and less in the production of health or nutrition? Does the intensity of agricultural labor increase or decrease? To what extent does this offset or magnify the beneficial effects that these changes may have on household income?

Third, are the inputs into health and nutrition complements or substitutes? If a certain level of nutritional status can be maintained by reducing time spent preparing meals and purchasing prepared foods, then these purchased foods are a substitute for time spent cooking. But not all inputs are substitutable. If a child is suffering from diarrhea, trying to increase her food consumption without treating the illness will not improve nutritional status.

Finally, how are these changes — their benefits and costs — distributed within the household and across households? Are the people who benefit from these changes the same people who incur costs?

Implications for Policy

These myriad links — both beneficial and adverse — among agriculture, health, and nutrition pose challenges for policymakers. In an area of ongoing research such as nutrition, the key policy lever for poor countries — where a large proportion of the population relies on agriculture for their livelihoods — will be the changes in crops, farm practices, and markets. Technological improvements and value-chain enhancements, if distributed effectively, can affect the supply of healthy and nutritious foods while simultaneously boosting incomes. It is this potential that makes agricultural innovation a leverage point for policy and programmatic interventions.

Concluding Remarks

The links among agriculture, health, and nutrition are most complex when we consider smallholder households. However, the framework is equally applicable to other household types. For example, landless rural households and urban households are typically net food consumers, and so changes in agriculture affect health and nutrition largely through changes in the quality, variety, and prices of foods available to them. The framework can also be readily adapted to national or global levels.

Anything that affects agriculture has the potential to affect health and nutrition, and anything that affects health and nutrition has the potential to affect agriculture. While some of these pathways imply that changes in agriculture will have positive impacts on human health, this is not true of all pathways. Policymakers in all sectors need to be cognizant of these multiple pathways and their bidirectional effects. The importance of different links will often be context-specific and determined by characteristics of the population being considered. The policy challenge is to ensure that changes occurring in agriculture come about in a way that maximizes benefits to human health and nutrition while minimizing the risks. Many of the chapters in this book describe particular contexts and circumstances where this has been achieved. Policy that uses the linkages among agriculture, health, and nutrition can produce good outcomes on all fronts.

Chapter 3

The Food System and Its Interaction with Human Health and Nutrition

Per Pinstrup-Andersen

The food system begins and ends with health and nutrition. Advances in the health sciences, including genomics and stem cell biology, continue to reinforce the principle that nutritious food is essential for the achievement of full physical and cognitive potential for all individuals and populations and for sustaining health through the aging process. Likewise, advances in the social and behavioral sciences are revealing the many dimensions of health, the behaviors that promote health, and the value of health in generating productive agricultural systems and sustainable development. Health is now considered a primary goal and quantifiable endpoint of food systems. It is also an important force in agricultural policy, driven in part by the emergence of the "triple burden" of malnutrition — the coexistence of hunger, nutrient deficiencies, and excess intake of calories leading to overweight and obesity in many poor countries — that has resulted in part from a lack of harmony between food systems and the promotion of human health.

Traditionally, an invisible firewall has separated the agriculture, health, and nutrition sectors. In university-level training and research, for example, health training, research, and projects reside in one part of the university, and agricultural training, research, and projects reside in another. This firewall extends to development organizations and governments' single-sector ministries. Yet evidence suggests that agricultural projects would have a greater health and nutritional impact if health and nutrition goals were explicitly integrated into their design and implementation. Indeed, one would expect strong interactions and synergies between health and nutrition and other parts of the food system — not just agriculture. An integrated approach to developing agriculture and food systems and improving health and nutrition would yield more effective and efficient solutions in all of these areas.

This chapter is based on *The African Food System and Its Interaction with Human Health and Nutrition,* ed. Per Pinstrup-Andersen (Ithaca, NY, US: Cornell University Press in cooperation with the United Nations University).

An Overview of the Food System, Health, and Nutrition

A food system may be described simply as a process that turns natural and human-made resources and inputs into food. As shown in Figure 1, such a system may consist of the resources (such as land, water, a healthy workforce, and sunshine); inputs (such as plant nutrients, pest-control measures, and knowledge); primary agricultural production; secondary production or processing; and transport, storage, and exchange activities to make the food available at the time and place and in the form desired by consumers. Food systems need not be stagnant. In fact, if the goal is to improve them, it is useful to visualize food systems as dynamic behavioral systems that can change in response to changes in the behavior of the various decisionmakers and agents within them, such as consumers, producers, market agents, resource owners, nongovernmental organizations, and governments.

Food systems are means to an end rather than ends in themselves. They exist to serve people. Their relations to human health and nutrition are many and strong, and they offer tremendous opportunities for improving or harming people's well-being—opportunities that need to be fully understood and acted upon. Food systems are also closely tied to natural resources and the climate, and the sustainability of food systems and improved health and nutrition depend on the health of the natural environment.

Each of the food-system activities may interact with health and nutrition, and Figure 2 illustrates some of these interactions. The most obvious interaction is

Figure 1   A food system

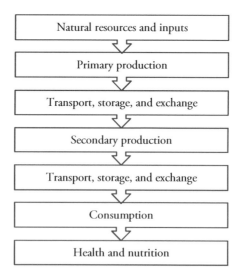

Source: Author.

FIgure 2 i nteractions between food systems and human health

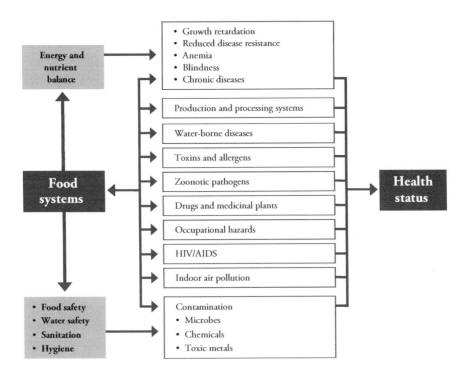

Source: Author.

the way in which the food system makes food available to meet people's needs for dietary energy and nutrients. Yet to achieve food security, individuals must have access to the food available, and their access is influenced by their purchasing power, their own production, and other factors. The food system may increase people's access through lower food prices brought about by lower unit costs of production, higher incomes among farmers and farm workers, and higher incomes outside the agricultural sector resulting from income-multiplier effects generated by higher farm incomes. Furthermore, changes in the food system may influence other determinants of nutrition, such as access to clean water and sanitation. Thus, changes in food systems may improve or worsen the nutrition situation, with repercussions on other health factors. It is estimated, for example, that more than half of developing countries' child mortality is associated with malnutrition and hunger. Children who suffer from hunger or malnutrition are less resistant to several infectious diseases and more likely to die from such illnesses. The food system may also contribute to increasing or decreasing the prevalence of chronic diseases by influencing changes in the prevalence of overweight and obesity.

Although much past research and debate have focused on the impact of agriculture on nutrition, it is important to recognize that there is a two-way causal relationship. Health and nutrition may also affect agriculture and food systems. For instance, energy and nutritional deficiencies, infectious diseases, obesity, and chronic diseases may influence food systems by lowering the labor productivity of food system workers; by reducing the adoption of improved technology and the use of inputs and credit; and by leading to suboptimal use of land, water, and other resources. Labor productivity may also be influenced by infectious diseases, such as malaria and bacterial and virus contamination, associated with water management in the food system.

Improving food quality in ways that support human health will require an integrated approach that encompasses both the agriculture and health sectors and will open new avenues of agricultural research. It will require coordinated efforts in the study of soil quality, plant varieties, crop and food engineering, food safety, climate change, plant and animal health, and food processing, among others. And because such an approach will require more diversity in the types of crops grown, with implications for all aspects of farming, it will raise new challenges for efforts to achieve sustainable agriculture.

The Poverty/Hunger/Ill-Health Trap

The interactions between agriculture, health, and nutrition mean that all three sectors play a role in the poverty/hunger/ill-health trap that afflicts millions of poor people around the world. Ultra-poverty (living on less than half a dollar a day), poor health, hunger, and malnutrition are mutually reinforcing conditions that push people into a poverty trap—a "self-reinforcing mechanism that causes poverty to persist" (Azariadis and Stachurski 2007). Widespread hunger and malnutrition combine with prevalent infectious diseases to cause poor health. Poor health and health shocks in turn have economic and productivity implications that are particularly pronounced in rural areas, where the food system is the main source of income and employment. In fact, recent research suggests that major health shocks may be the leading cause of collapse into long-term poverty. The productivity consequences of health shocks are likely to be most severe for farmers and others who undertake hard physical work. Furthermore, the income effects of health shocks will be direct and severe among semi-subsistence farmers, who may not be able to provide the labor needed to bring the crop to harvest. The resulting poverty trap has dire implications for human well-being, cognitive development, and individual and national incomes.

The prevalence of poverty traps points to the importance of strategies that integrate health, food, nutrition, and environment. Christopher Barrett (2010) has noted that "all past cases of rapid, widespread progress out of poverty have been causally associated with the transformation of food systems."

An Integrated Approach

The interactions between the food system and human health and nutrition illustrated in Figure 2 point to several potential areas for integrated action that can serve the goals of all three sectors.

- *Biofortification.* Efforts to develop and diffuse nutritionally fortified food crops offer very promising opportunities for reducing micronutrient deficiencies in a sustainable manner. Industrial fortification may help reduce such deficiencies in urban areas and rural areas with highly developed infrastructure. A more effective avenue for reaching nutrient-deficient people in most rural areas of developing countries to alter the seeds so that staple food crops consumed by low-income people may contain more absorbable nutrients.

- *Zoonotic diseases.* Many of the health problems affecting humans—including measles, tuberculosis, AIDS, avian and swine influenza, and mad cow disease—originated with animals. A better understanding of disease transmission mechanisms and extensive surveillance for early detection of disease outbreaks could help strengthen both agricultural systems and human health. E. Fuller Torrey (2011) points out that four other factors will also require attention: (1) the relationship between animals and humans and reconsideration of the sharing of living space; (2) modes of transportation that facilitate transmission of infectious diseases; (3) animal slaughter practices and other food-processing activities; and (4) ecological and environmental shifts such as urbanization, climate change, and deforestation.

- *HIV/AIDS.* In parts of Africa, food insecurity and HIV/AIDS coexist and interact in a vicious circle. Agricultural policies and programs that are responsive to this can further both AIDS-related goals and agricultural productivity goals. Collaboration among nutritionists, agricultural economists, and program managers could enhance programs designed to improve food security for households and communities (Gillespie 2010).

- *Crop protection.* Better agroecological pest management in agriculture could help reduce pesticide use and thereby protect farmers from exposure to excessive pesticides and consumers from toxins in the food supply. An integrated crop-management approach would consider crop diversity and resiliency and incorporate host-plant tolerance and resistance when possible, relying on chemical pesticides as a last resort (Nelson 2010).

• *Sustainable management of natural resources.* Agriculture, nutrition, and health all have important links to the natural environment. Unsustainable management of land, water, and other natural resources can lead to soil erosion, siltation in watersheds, seasonal water scarcities, and water-borne and insect vector–transmitted diseases, with negative effects on agricultural yields and incomes as well as on nutrition and health. In contrast, sustainable management of land and water and preservation of biodiversity can help improve health and nutrition not only directly but also indirectly by maintaining agricultural yields and incomes (Herforth 2010).

• *Food safety.* Given the weak food control systems, poor infrastructure, lack of resources, and improper food handling common in many developing countries, food- and water-borne diseases impose a high burden on poor people, yet they are often overlooked, unreported, or ignored. Improvements should be made to food safety along the entire food chain, from production to storage, transportation, and processing. Also needed are improvements in surveillance systems and in public awareness of basic hygiene and food safety measures. It is important to recognize, however, that if improving food safety raises the cost of food, it may threaten the food security of the poorest people (Nakimbugwe and Boor 2010).

These kinds of integrated approaches, as well as other poverty-reducing policies that promote agricultural productivity, improve rural infrastructure, and strengthen domestic markets, will help create sustainable health and nutrition improvements.

Approaches like these, however, take time to show impact. In the short term, complementary programs and policies, such as income and transfer programs and primary healthcare, are needed (Alderman 2010). Many poor people who suffer from chronic hunger, malnutrition, and health problems are defenseless against income shocks caused by production, market, or employment losses. Without safety nets or some other insurance mechanism, income shocks can result in severe suffering, further nutrition and health deterioration, and death. Safety net programs, and the mechanisms to target them to beneficiaries, need to be context-specific and take into account what is known about how households behave, including how household decisionmaking relates to gender (see Box 1). It is important to view such programs not as unproductive handouts, but as investments in human resources and future economic growth and stability. Not only are health and nutrition intrinsically

---

BOx 1 e   mpower w omen to Play an effective r ole

The link between health and productivity is particularly important for women—partly because of the role women play in food production, food preparation, and child care and partly because of their special vulnerabilities related to reproductive health. The limited communication between agricultural and health research is an obstacle to women's ability to meet nutrition and health goals for themselves and their families.

Women are key players in food systems—in Africa, for instance, they account for 70 percent of farm labor and perform 80 percent of food processing. They are certain to play a large role in producing increased food supplies to meet rising demand. But women must be given the power to play their role in agriculture effectively. They will require access to land rights, water-use rights, credit, extension services, and well-functioning markets for inputs and outputs. In many areas women smallholder farmers are attempting to raise their incomes through better access to output markets, and supermarkets are offering new market opportunities. But these opportunities also present smallholders with new competitive conditions, requirements for improved food safety, and demands for consistency in quantity and quality, which they may have difficulties meeting.

Agricultural projects and policies must therefore take context-specific gender norms and women's heavy time demands and constraints into account. Both women and men should be involved in developing priorities and implementation strategies for projects and research for the food system (Cramer and Wandira 2010).

---

important measures of well-being, but they can make workers more productive and thereby help transform food systems into vehicles for greater economic growth and poverty alleviation.

The Bottom Line

Human health and nutrition are both the foundation of a strong food system and the expected outcome from such a system. An integrated multidisciplinary systems approach to research and development in human health and the food system, with due consideration to natural environment issues, thus offers great advantages over single-sector approaches, irrespective of whether the goal is improved health, improved nutrition, improved food systems, or sustainable management of the natural environment. In fact, the achievement of all four goals can be pursued in a systems approach. Any trade-offs among them can be explicitly identified and assessed, and double, triple, and quadruple wins are possible. Given the new awareness of the strong interactive relationships that exist among health, the food system, and the natural environment, existing firewalls between them should be broken down so that the advantages of an integrated systems approach can come into play for the world's poor and hungry people.

r eferences

Alderman, H. 2010. "Income and Food Transfers to Improve Human Health and Nutrition." In *The African Food System and Its Interaction with Human Health and Nutrition*, edited by P. Pinstrup-Andersen. Ithaca, NY, US: Cornell University Press in cooperation with the United Nations University.

Azariadis, C., and J. Stachurski. 2007. "Poverty Traps." In *Handbook of Economic Growth*, edited by P. Aghion and S. Durlauf, vol. 1B. Amsterdam, the Netherlands: Elsevier, 33.

Barrett, C. 2010. "Food Systems and the Escape from Poverty and Ill-Health Traps in Sub-Saharan Africa." In *The African Food System and Its Interaction with Human Health and Nutrition*, edited by P. Pinstrup-Andersen. Ithaca, NY, US: Cornell University Press in cooperation with the United Nations University.

Cramer, L. K., and S. K. Wandira. 2010. "Strengthening the Role of Women in the Food Systems of Sub-Saharan Africa to Achieve Nutrition and Health Goals." In *The African Food System and Its Interaction with Human Health and Nutrition*, edited by P. Pinstrup-Andersen. Ithaca, NY, US: Cornell University Press in cooperation with the United Nations University.

Gillespie, S. 2010. "How AIDS Epidemics Interact with African Food Systems and How to Improve the Response." In *The African Food System and Its Interaction with Human Health and Nutrition*, edited by P. Pinstrup-Andersen. Ithaca, NY, US: Cornell University Press in cooperation with the United Nations University.

Herforth, A. 2010. "Nutrition and the Environment: Fundamental to Food Security in Africa." In *The African Food System and Its Interaction with Human Health and Nutrition*, edited by P. Pinstrup-Andersen. Ithaca, NY, US: Cornell University Press in cooperation with the United Nations University.

Nakimbugwe, D., and K. J. Boor. 2010. "Food Safety as a Bridge between the Food System and Human Health in Sub-Saharan Africa." In *The African Food System and Its Interaction with Human Health and Nutrition*, edited by P. Pinstrup-Andersen. Ithaca, NY, US: Cornell University Press in cooperation with the United Nations University.

Nelson, R. 2010. "Pest Management, Farmer Incomes, and Health Risks in Sub- Saharan Africa: Pesticides, Host Plant Resistance, and Other Measures," in *The African Food System and Its Interaction with Human Health and Nutrition*, edited by P. Pinstrup-Andersen. Ithaca, NY, US: Cornell University Press in cooperation with the United Nations University.

Pinstrup-Andersen, P. and D. D. Watson. 2011. *Food Policy for Developing Countries: The Role of Government in Global, National, and Local Food Systems.* Ithaca, NY, US: Cornell University Press in cooperation with the United Nations University.

Torrey, E. F. 2010. "Animals as a Source of Human Diseases: Historical Perspective and Future Health Risks for the African Population." In *The African Food System and Its Interaction with Human Health and Nutrition*, edited by P. Pinstrup-Andersen. Ithaca, NY, US: Cornell University Press in cooperation with the United Nations University.

Chapter 4

The Nexus between Agriculture and Nutrition: Do Growth Patterns and Conditional Factors Matter?

Shenggen Fan and Joanna Brzeska

Although tremendous progress has been made in meeting the world's food demand, many parts of the developing world suffer from undernutrition—that is, deficiencies in energy, protein, and essential vitamins and minerals. Economic growth, which many assume has a naturally positive impact on people's nutritional status through increased incomes and food expenditures has not translated into improved nutrition in a number of developing countries. The 2007–08 food price crisis and the recent food price increase have pushed millions of people into hunger, indicating how vulnerable the poor are to shocks in production and markets.

As part of overall economic growth, agricultural growth has an especially important role to play in reducing and preventing undernutrition through a number of channels. Its impact extends from increased household ability to purchase and produce more nutritious food to economywide effects, such as lowering food prices and increasing government revenues to fund health, infrastructure, and nutrition intervention programs. Questions remain, however, about the effects of different patterns of agricultural growth on nutrition. Furthermore, other factors—such as infrastructure, the status of women (including their education level), income and land distribution, and access to resources and services—may contribute to how well agricultural growth translates into nutritional improvements.

This chapter examines how different growth patterns lead to different nutritional outcomes and identifies the factors that influence the magnitude of this relationship. It aims to offer researchers insights on areas for future research and analysis and provide policymakers with potential development strategies and investment policies that will increase the likelihood of positive nutritional outcomes.

This chapter is based on the authors' 2020 Conference Paper, *The Nexus between Agriculture and Nutrition: Do Growth Patterns and Conditional Factors Matter?* (Washington, DC: International Food Policy Research Institute, 2011).

Does Growth Matter?

Few studies have tried to explain and quantify how economic growth contributes to reducing undernutrition. One reason could be the widely accepted assumption that economic growth will ultimately lead to improved nutrition through increased incomes and food expenditures. However, the limited evidence that exists offers either inconclusive or conflicting results on the link between growth and nutrition.

A number of studies find that overall economic growth—usually represented by gross domestic product (GDP), per capita GDP, and per capita income—is only weakly associated with indicators of nutritional status and argue instead in favor of more direct nutrition interventions (Neeliah and Shankar 2008). In contrast, another group of studies has found a positive and significant link between increased economic growth and nutritional status—either unidirectional or bidirectional (Subramanian and Deaton 2009). One cross-country study, for example, not only found that income growth had a positive effect on children's weight-for-age but also projected that similar income growth rates can produce significantly different reductions in malnutrition across countries over a period of about 25 years (Haddad et al. 2003). (See Figure 1.) Because many of these countries have not been able to sustain significant annual income growth, the authors argue that improving nutritional status will require balancing income growth with cost-effective health and nutrition interventions, including vitamin supplementation and nutrition education.

FiGure 1   Projected reduction in child malnutrition rate with 2.5 percent annual growth in per capita income, 1990s to 2015

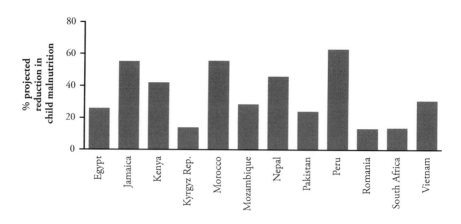

Source: Haddad et al. 2003.

Discrepancies in the findings of past growth–nutrition studies are commonly attributed to a number of shortcomings: poor-quality data that are often not comparable across countries, failure to recognize the nonlinear and dynamic relationship between growth and nutrition, and disregard for issues related to diet quality resulting from different patterns of growth. These limitations support the argument that growth and nutrition are not homogenous entities and should not be treated as such.

Do Sectoral Growth Patterns Matter?

Past experience has shown that agricultural development can serve as an engine of growth and poverty reduction, primarily for two reasons: (1) there are backward and forward links in production and consumption between agriculture and the rest of the economy, and (2) the majority of poor people live in rural areas, so agriculture makes up a large share of their income, expenditures, and employment. The question we face now is to what extent can agricultural growth—and growth in particular subsectors of agriculture—be a springboard for nutritional improvement through such channels as increased agricultural production and lower food prices.

Although empirical evidence on the nutritional impacts of agricultural growth is limited, it shows that the impact varies across measures of undernutrition and stages of development. One cross-country study finds that agricultural growth, in particular, is associated with a reduction in underweight and leads to reduced stunting in more food-insecure countries, with the exception of India (Headey 2011). While evidence from the analysis also suggests that the effect of agricultural growth on calorie intake is significant, its effect on diet diversity—used as a rough proxy for micronutrient consumption—is minimal. A study conducted in Yemen shows that although agricultural growth can lead to large reductions in undernutrition, its impact on stunting is only about 10 percent of its impact on calorie deficiency (Ecker, Breisinger, and Pauw 2011). Furthermore, cross-country evidence from the study shows that the growth–nutrition relationship varies according to a country's economic status, with the largest impact occurring at low levels of per capita GDP.

Within the agriculture sector, individual subsectors—like staple crops or livestock—have different impacts on development outcomes. Whether growth in a subsector is pro-poor and pro-nutrition depends on (1) its linkages with the rest of the economy, (2) its initial size and geographic concentration, (3) its growth potential, and (4) market opportunities. A study in Tanzania, for example, found that high agricultural growth did little to improve nutrition because it was driven primarily by crops less likely to be grown by the poor (Pauw and Thurlow 2010). Other studies have also found that growth in staple crops contributes more to poverty reduction and calorie intake than does growth in export crops, given that poor farmers often lack the financial resources and technologies to cultivate crops for export. These differences in the impacts of agricultural subsectors are amplified by regional variations in natural resources and economic conditions in many developing countries, so maximizing the potential of specific agricultural subsectors to improve nutrition requires regionally differentiated strategies.

Policymakers can thus boost the effectiveness of growth—in terms of poverty reduction and improved calorie and micronutrient intake—by seeking to accelerate growth with stronger links to specific population groups and regions and to specific subsectors like vegetables, fruits, and livestock. Research on the effects of different growth patterns on nutrition needs to go beyond calorie intake to include a range of indicators of nutritional status, including micronutrient intake and wasting, underweight, and stunting among children.

How Do Conditional Factors Affect the Links between Growth and Nutrition Outcomes?

A number of factors related to underlying conditions affect the links between growth and nutrition outcomes. Given the same rate of economic or agricultural growth, improvements in these conditional factors will result in better nutrition outcomes, whereas the lack of attention to these factors can result in growth having a smaller impact on nutrition.

Equity in income and access to resources and services: High income inequality, unequal allocation of productive assets (such as land and water), and unequal access to health and education services within developing countries have been linked to lower nutritional status. Income inequality, for example, is associated with a misdistribution of food that results in the overconsumption of food by privileged groups and food insecurity among poor people. More equal access to health and education services is vital for human capital formation through channels such as increased nutrition knowledge and income-generation skills. Similarly, more egalitarian land endowments provide a greater number of individuals and households with a source of income and facilitate farm households' access to food from their own production, which is especially important in areas with underdeveloped markets. In fact, one of the main features distinguishing China from other developing countries with high growth and high malnutrition rates—such as India—is China's relatively egalitarian distribution of land, virtual lack of landlessness, and relatively equal access to health and education services.

Women's status: Gender inequality in nutrition—resulting from women's weak land rights; lower levels of education; and lack of access to credit, extension services, and technologies—has been widely documented, especially in South Asia. However, many past growth–nutrition analyses have overlooked the potential impact of gender-based variables. When women have more control over household resources and better access to health services and education, child and household nutrition rates have been found to be higher. In fact, low-income female-headed households often exhibit better nutrition than higher-income male-headed households. While agricultural growth that benefits women can lead to improved household and child nutritional status through higher incomes among women, it can also have a negative impact on nutrition by changing time and labor allocation patterns, which reduces women's time for child care and the quality of food provided by the mother.

Rural infrastructure: A large body of evidence has closely linked investment in infrastructure—including roads, water, sanitation, and electricity—with growth in agricultural productivity and poverty reduction, and infrastructure is also positively related to better nutrition through a variety of channels. Improved infrastructure can promote income growth by raising agricultural productivity, lowering production and transaction costs, and removing bottlenecks that impede the participation of the poor in the development process, thereby facilitating increased access to, availability of, and consumption of food among larger segments of the population. It also improves people's access to more and better healthcare and sanitation services. A number of studies in countries such as India, Peru, and Sudan have found a positive association between the quality and quantity of infrastructure development and nutritional status. However, evidence also shows that the magnitude—and, at times, even the existence—of the nutritional impact of improved infrastructure differs across population groups.

Health status: Health and nutritional status are directly linked through a synergistic relationship. Illness impairs nutritional status by reducing both appetite and the ability of the body to absorb nutrients, which in turn lowers the individual's resistance to further illness. Health status can also have a significant impact on nutrition by affecting a household's ability to take part in productive activities that generate food or income to purchase food. Working through these pathways, sickness and death have been shown to result in a reduction of cultivated land, food production, and crop varieties. Absenteeism and the loss of labor resulting from ill health can lead to changes in cropping patterns and declines in crop diversity, with affected households switching to less labor-intensive crops—such as root crops—that are often lower in nutritional value.

Strategies and investments for Pro-Nutrition Growth

Given the dynamic relationship between agricultural growth and nutritional status, nutritional improvements can be addressed in a number of ways. The question is how to set priorities and allocate limited public resources.

Growth Strategy

The relationship between growth (whether nonagricultural or agricultural) and nutrition is not straightforward, and more solid research is needed to support evidence-based policymaking and strategy formulation. For growth strategies to maximize their effect on nutrition, the different impacts of specific economic and agricultural policies and conditional factors on growth–nutrition links need to be taken into account. So far, nutrition has not been widely used as an objective of economic or agricultural growth strategies. Food and nutrition fall under several government entities (including ministries of agriculture, social affairs, and health), with the result that nutrition is often a political and institutional orphan. It is thus difficult to incorporate nutrition effectively into a country's main agricultural strategy, which is designed mostly by the ministry of agriculture.

Growth strategies need to be designed with a nutritional lens and should take into account what types of sectoral and subsectoral practices and policies can enhance nutrition. These strategies could include the following:

- promoting productivity growth of more nutritious foods to increase food supplies and reduce high and volatile food prices;

- increasing demand for and access to nutritious foods along the entire value chain through consumer knowledge and awareness campaigns;

- mitigating health and nutrition risks associated with agriculture, such as water-borne, food-borne, and zoonotic diseases as well as occupational injuries and health hazards; and

- breeding more nutritious varieties of staple food crops that are consumed by poor people in developing countries through biofortification initiatives, such as the HarvestPlus Challenge Program of the CGIAR.

Setting priorities and sequencing such interventions as part of a pro-nutrition growth strategy will depend on country-specific conditions, stages of development, and institutional capacity.

investment Strategy and Fiscal Policies

Public investments in rural infrastructure and agricultural research have been shown to have one of the largest impacts on poverty reduction and economic growth in a number of developing countries. There is no empirical evidence, however, showing how different types of public spending affect nutrition. Given that public resources in most developing countries are scarce and the opportunity cost is high, decisionmakers should seek to allocate public resources more efficiently. This means taking into account the positive and negative spillover effects on nutrition and comparing them to other development outcomes, such as poverty reduction. Research on the effects of public investment should be expanded to include nutrition in order to give policymakers information on how to prioritize public spending according to nutritional and other development outcomes.

Fiscal policies, like taxes on unhealthy foods and subsidies on nutrient-rich foods, can also be used to maximize positive and minimize negative spillover effects on nutrition. While taxes on foods rich in saturated fats can be useful in generating government revenue, studies in developed countries show that such policies need to be complemented by interventions that discourage the consumption of these foods, including subsidies on nutrient-rich foods such as fruits and vegetables. More research is needed on the impacts of these kinds of policies in developing countries.

Conclusion

A new paradigm for agricultural development is needed, whereby agricultural growth leads not only to increased production and reduced poverty but also to improved nutrition. The need for a new paradigm is especially pressing in light of rising food prices and stubbornly high rates of hunger and malnutrition. The question facing many developing countries is how to set priorities and sequence interventions to maximize the benefits from the dynamic and nonlinear relationship between growth and nutrition while also paying attention to the role of conditional factors. Growth, particularly agricultural growth, is still necessary to push down food prices, thus enabling the majority of the poor and hungry to benefit. The recent food crisis has clearly shown that the poor are especially sensitive to changes in food prices.

Growth alone, however, is not sufficient to address undernutrition. It is thus also important to identify the likely trade-offs between implementing pro-nutrition growth strategies, pursuing other objectives such as poverty reduction, and using instruments such as targeted nutrition programs—continuously paying extra attention to the distribution of benefits and costs across different population groups.

To help policymakers make sound decisions about priorities and sequencing, more research is needed on the impact of different sectoral patterns and public investment policies on nutrition and how this impact varies across different economic, geographic, and social conditions. This research needs to be based on more comprehensive nutrition data, including micronutrient intakes across different segments of the population.

Finally, strong institutions and governance, as well as monitoring and transparency, are vital to ensure that nutritional objectives are not left out of the development process and that pro-nutrition growth strategies and investment policies are effective.

r eferences

Ecker, O., C. Breisinger, and K. Pauw. 2011. "Linking Economic Policy to Nutrition Outcomes: Applications to Yemen and Malawi." Background paper for the conference "Leveraging Agriculture for Improving Nutrition and Health," organized by the International Food Policy Research Institute (IFPRI), New Delhi, February 10–12.

Haddad, L., H. Alderman, S. Appleton, L. Song, and Y. Yohannes. 2003. "Reducing Malnutrition: How Far Does Income Growth Take Us?" *World Bank Economic Review* 17 (1): 107–131.

Headey, D. 2011. "Turning Economic Growth into Nutrition-Sensitive Growth." Background paper for the conference "Leveraging Agriculture for Improving Nutrition and Health," organized by the International Food Policy Research Institute (IFPRI), New Delhi, February 10–12.

Neeliah, H., and B. Shankar. 2008. "Is Nutritional Improvement a Cause or a Consequence of Economic Growth? Evidence from Mauritius." *Economics Bulletin* 17 (8): 1–11.

O'Donnell, O., A. Nicolás, and E. Van Doorslaer. 2009. "Growing Richer and Taller: Explaining Change in the Distribution of Child Nutritional Status during Vietnam's Economic Boom." *Journal of Development Economics* 88 (1): 45–58.

Pauw, K., and J. Thurlow. 2010. *Agricultural Growth, Poverty, and Nutrition in Tanzania.* IFPRI Discussion Paper 947. Washington, DC: International Food Policy Research Institute.

Subramanian, S., and A. Deaton, 1996. "The Demand for Food and Calories." *Journal of Political Economy* 104 (1): 133–162.

Chapter 5

Turning Economic Growth into Nutrition-Sensitive Growth

Derek Headey

There is a growing consensus that reducing childhood malnutrition is a critically important goal, but there is far less agreement on what strategies can best achieve that goal. Are more nutrition-specific interventions required, such as food and nutrient supplements or training and education programs? Or does the answer lie in broader social developments such as rising incomes, increased food security, and better access to education, health, infrastructure, and family planning services? These factors can all be seen as facets of integrated socioeconomic development, but stakeholders rightly point to examples of economic growth leading to little or no reduction in childhood malnutrition. This does not rule out an important role for economic growth, however, provided that its benefits translate into increased food availability, reductions in poverty, and broader social development—that economic growth is "nutrition-sensitive."

The Impact of Economic Growth on Nutrition

There is no existing literature that explicitly tests whether these elements of nutrition-sensitive growth really have a large impact on changes in malnutrition over the medium term. Existing research is either country specific or it only focuses on long-term questions, such as why malnutrition rates change across regions (space), rather than across time (Smith and Haddad 2000; Heltberg 2009; Webb and Block 2010). This bolsters the need for a dynamic cross-country approach that explains changes in malnutrition over the medium term, which is more consistent with the question of how to achieve the Millennium Development Goals (MDGs). And in addition to deriving "on average" results, there is also a need to systematically examine the role of economic growth in particular countries. The data can then be used to analyze successes and failures in the war against malnutrition.

This chapter is based on the author's 2020 Conference Paper, *Turning Economic Growth into Nutrition-Sensitive Growth* (Washington, DC: International Food Policy Research Institute, 2011).

Box 1   Data and Methods

Research data for the examination in this chapter come from several sources, which were mined, compared, and cross- referenced to provide a rich collection of indicators, outcomes, and trends. These sources include the Demographic and Health Surveys (DHS), the World Bank's World Development Index, and Agrostat (from the Food and Agriculture Organization of the United Nations).

With regard to malnutrition indicators, this chapter focuses on the prevalence of stunting (low height-for-age), since this is the best measure of the cumulative effects of various malnutrition processes (such as dietary deficiencies and exposure to infectious diseases). However, the conference paper upon which this chapter is based also tests the sensitivity of results to the use of underweight prevalence and low BMI prevalence for adult women.

Productive Sector Dimensions of Nutrition-Sensitive Growth: A Special Role for Agriculture?

Does overall economic growth explain reductions in malnutrition? And, if so, do the sources of that growth— agricultural or nonagricultural—produce different effects on malnutrition? Statistical tests reveal the following:

First, general economic growth—in gross domestic product (GDP) per capita— predicts reductions in stunting, and the effect is reasonably large. A per capita GDP growth rate of 5.0 percent per year predicts a reduction in national stunting prevalence of around 0.9 percentage point per year. In the longer term, a doubling of GDP per capita would predict a reduction of around 18.0 percentage points. These effects are sizeable, but they also show a lot of variation around the mean: growth leads to reductions in stunting in many but not all cases. This suggests that the sources of growth might matter.

Second, agricultural growth has a large and significant effect in reducing stunting, but only outside of India, where a third of the world's malnourished children reside. Outside of India, agricultural growth appears to lead to larger reductions in stunting than nonagricultural growth, although the impact of agricultural growth is conditional upon the size of the sector. For example, agricultural growth would be very important for reducing malnutrition in an agrarian economy like Ethiopia, but much less important in an industrial economy such as Singapore. In Indian states, however, there is no evidence that agricultural growth has reduced stunting in recent decades. A stark example is the state of Gujarat, which has experienced extremely rapid agricultural and nonagricultural growth without any significant reductions in malnutrition.

Third, increased food production seems to be the most important linkage between agricultural growth and nutrition. Tests show that increased agricultural growth has a very large effect on average calorie availability, especially when initial calorie availability is low. However, nonagricultural growth seems to have larger effects on dietary diversity. This is consistent with the idea that poor economies first fulfill their basic calorie requirements through domestic food production (since many food staples are basically nontradable), before rising incomes eventually lead to more diverse diets.

Social Dimensions of Nutrition-Sensitive Growth: A Nutrition-Sensitive Social Development Index (NUSSDI)

While the source of economic growth matters, it is also important to consider how the benefits of growth are used for social sector development. A large amount of survey-based literature has uncovered significant associations between nutrition outcomes and a range of policy-related social sector outcomes. To see which outcomes systematically explain changes in stunting in a cross-country setting, a range of variables were tested with a view to constructing an index. The strongest relationships hold for four variables: (1) a poverty proxy (ownership of at least one asset), (2) a health proxy (medically attended births), (3) a female education proxy (women's secondary and tertiary education), and (4) a family planning proxy (fertility rates). Infrastructure variables—such as improved water, sanitation, and electricity access—show weak relationships, although they could still be important as parts of an overall development strategy that includes a focus on malnutrition.

The four strongest variables neatly capture several different determinants of malnutrition and may be good proxies for broader socioeconomic dimensions that are relevant to nutrition outcomes, such as gender empowerment (female education and fertility rates), birth spacing and age at marriage (fertility rates), and overall health access (medically attended births). Hence the final nutrition-sensitive social development index (NUSSDI) is an equally weighted sum of these four variables, and it ranges between 0 and 100.

This index and its components can be used to answer two questions. First, are improvements in NUSSDI scores as powerful a determinant of reductions in stunting as general economic growth? Second, does economic growth drive changes in NUSSDI scores? In answer to the first question, there is evidence that improvements in NUSSDI scores have larger effects on stunting than commensurate increases in GDP per capita. In answer to the second question, the results suggest that economic growth has positive effects on all four components of NUSSDI. For example, the estimates suggest that a doubling of GDP per capita would increase women's secondary education by 14 percentage points and access to medical births by 18 percentage points. The effects on asset-based poverty are somewhat weak, although this may be because this measure pertains to extreme poverty. So, in general, economic growth does typically bring about significant changes in these four dimensions of socioeconomic development but with large variations across different growth episodes.

Successes and Failures

While formal tests suggest that nutrition-sensitive development typically requires increased food production along with broader socioeconomic developments, it is important to verify these findings with actual country experiences. To do so the study identifies the most successful and least successful nutrition episodes in the dataset in terms of changes in both stunting and underweight prevalence, as the former was not always available. The criteria for success are twofold. First, a country (or Indian state) must show progress against at least one childhood malnutrition indicator faster than 1 percentage point per year. As it happens, this minimum speed of progress would almost always ensure success in meeting the MDG target of halving malnutrition in 25 years, unless initial malnutrition prevalence was well above 50 percent. Second, there must at least be some progress against the other childhood malnutrition indicator (in other words, a country or state cannot show progress on one front but regress on another). As for the definition of failure, it is defined as a 0.4 percent per year increase in at least one childhood malnutrition variable, and no progress on the other.

For each of these case studies, trends in the determinants of nutrition-sensitive development were also documented, including whether the episode was accompanied by rapid economic growth (including in agriculture), increased food availability, and improvements in the four dimensions of NUSSDI. Finally, successes and failures were further categorized into various groups, such as "proven" and "unproven" successes. Proven successes mostly include longer episodes where there were also nutrition-specific programs in place, whereas unproven successes refer to recent episodes that have not yet stood the test of time.

Do the success stories and failures confirm the more formal statistical findings? The short answer is yes, although there are some important caveats.

For example, among the "proven" success stories, relatively strong economic growth—including growth in agricultural production—is prominent. The only significant exceptions to this conclusion are middle-income countries like Brazil and Mexico in the 1980s and Honduras in the late 1990s, where it appears that existing national income was high enough to fund effective social development programs.

In all other cases—like Bangladesh, Tamil Nadu, Thailand, and Vietnam—there was quite rapid economic growth, as well as broader socioeconomic developments and nutrition- specific programs in place. The combination of significant agriculture growth and improved social development outcomes is also evident for most Green Revolution episodes (characterized by rapid growth in cereal production) as well as the vast majority of "unproven" success stories, albeit with two important exceptions. First, reductions in fertility only feature prominently in the longer-term "proven" success stories. Second, dietary changes show only a weak association with success against malnutrition, although this may be because of measurement error (national food availability is measured rather than the food intake of children or mothers) and because initial dietary conditions vary across countries (in some countries food availability is a problem, in others less so). (See Table 1.)

In terms of failures, a number of episodes in which malnutrition increased are explained by conflict, extreme governance failures, or decreased food availability. But much more puzzling examples of nutrition failures also occur in environments of strong economic growth, including Egypt, Gujarat, and Kazakhstan. The success stories therefore suggest that while nutrition-sensitive economic growth may well be a necessary condition for sustained reductions in malnutrition in low-income countries, economic growth is not a sufficient condition for nutritional improvements.

Key Findings

This chapter asks if nutrition-sensitive economic growth is an effective strategy for reducing malnutrition, and what that kind of growth looks like. To answer these questions, the author drew on rigorous statistical tests in which productive and social sector outcomes have the most impact on reductions in malnutrition. As with all findings, there are caveats, but the following results are nevertheless intuitive and well supported by the available evidence.

First, r apid e conomic g rowth i s a n ecessary co ndition fo r s ustainably r educing malnutrition at lower levels of development. While the number of sustained success stories is small, there is no example yet of a low-income country significantly reducing malnutrition without longer-term economic growth.

Second, a gricultural g rowth w ill o ften h ave a l arger im pact o n m alnutrition than n onagricultural g rowth, b ut t his a dvantage is h ighly c onditional u pon the s ize of the sector, the extent to which food insecurity is a problem, and the extent to which agricultural growth delivers increased food availability. The main exception to this statement is that the result does not appear to apply in post-reform India (1992 onward), where around a third of the world's malnourished children reside. This warrants further investigation.

TABl E 1   Successful episodes in fighting malnutrition

episodes	change in underweight (points per year)	change in stunting (points per year)	Better diets (calories, proteins, fats)	growth >5%/year (agriculture >3%/year)	Favorable health, education, and fertility trends
Proven long-term successes with well-documented nutrition programs					
Bangladesh 1994–2005	−2.0	−2.0	Very rapid	Yes (agric.)	Yes
Brazil 1986–96	−0.7	−1.9	Yes	No	Yes (very rapid)
Honduras 1996–2001	−1.3	−1.8	Diversifying	No	Yes
Tamil Nadu 1992–98	−1.9	N.A.	Diversifying	Yes	Yes
Thailand 1982–90	−2.9	N.A.	Very rapid	Yes	Yes
Vietnam 1994–2006	−1.5	−1.3	Very rapid	Yes (agric.)	Yes
green r evolution episodes with marked increases in cereal production					
Bangladesh 1985–94	−1.1	N.A.	Very rapid	Yes (GDP=4.7%)	Yes
India 1977–92	−1.3	N.A.	Very rapid	Yes (agric.)	No (exc. fertility)
Philippines 1973–82	−1.9	N.A.	Yes (cereals)	Yes (agric.)	Yes (education)
Sri Lanka 1977–87	−1.8	−1.3	Yes (protein)	Yes (agric.)	Yes
unproven short-term successes					
Angola 1996–2001	−1.9	−2.2	Yes	Yes (agric.)	Yes (exc. fertility)
Cambodia 1996–2006	−1.4	−1.5	Yes	Yes (agric.)	Yes
Ethiopia 2000–05	−1.5	−1.3	Yes	Yes (agric.)	Only fertility
Ghana 2003–06	−1.6	−2.5	Yes	Yes (agric.)	Only education
Kyrgyzstan 1997–2006	−0.6	−1.6	Modest	No	Yes (exc. fertility)
Punjab 1992–98	−2.8	−1.5	No (decline)	Yes	Yes
Tanzania 1996–2005	−1.5	−0.6	Diversifying	Yes (agric.)	No
Uzbekistan 1996–2006	−1.1	−1.9	No	Yes (agric.)	Yes (exc. fertility)

Source: Author's construction.

Third, social sector outcomes are also critical components of nutrition-sensitive development. Cross-country evidence suggests that the most robust nutrition-sensitive elements of social sector development are poverty reduction and health, education, and family planning outcomes. Infrastructure investments may also be important, but the evidence thus far is somewhat weak. And as with overall economic growth, the analysis of successes and failures suggests that these kinds of investments are a necessary but not sufficient condition for sustained reductions in malnutrition.

The main caveats to these conclusions are measurement error and data availability. Data on the quality of diets are weak, and the sample of proven success stories is fairly small. Hence, it will be important to revisit these inferences in the light of new experiences. There are still no definitive answers as to why there appears to be an agriculture disconnect in India, although existing research suggests that there may in fact be multiple disconnects, with poverty, nutrition, education, health, and family planning policies all regarded as possible suspects.

To go about developing more nutrition-sensitive growth strategies, there are obviously important impediments that need to be overcome. *First, malnutrition is often misperceived by policymakers as a simple food problem, rather than a complex multisectoral problem.* Welcome efforts to raise awareness of the problem mostly focus on outcomes—such as the Global Hunger Index—but more emphasis is needed on monitoring inputs, including better tracking of more specific nutrition policies.

Second, researchers and policymakers need to encourage more cross-country learning. Despite notable success stories, remarkably few countries have large-scale multisectoral nutrition strategies in place, and there is consequently little evidence of cross-country learning. Yet two prominent examples show that it can be done. In Thailand, the main champions of the nutrition program came from health, education, and agriculture, and these champions pushed other policymakers into receiving nutrition education and training from overseas. Hence, it was possible to develop an integrated, multipronged approach. In Bangladesh, the learning was more explicit, since Bangladesh's Integrated Nutrition Program was adapted from Tamil Nadu's program. But these examples are far too few, suggesting it is essential for researchers to facilitate more cross-country learning, and for policymakers to provide the political impetus to translate knowledge into action.

Concluding Remarks

Results support the plausible hypothesis that economic growth reduces childhood malnutrition through five important channels: increased food availability, reductions in poverty, improvements in female education, increased access to health services, and improved family planning outcomes. Other channels may be important, such as improved infrastructure, but the cross-country evidence is thus far not strong.

The findings go to the heart of the debate about whether nutrition-specific strategies should be pursued, or whether broader development strategies suffice. This is partly a matter of perspective. In the short run, targeted nutrition interventions (for example, food, vitamin, or mineral supplements and education and training programs) could have high returns even in the absence of economic growth or broader social sector development. In the longer term, however, a nutrition-sensitive growth strategy is undoubtedly the best means of sustainably eradicating malnutrition. This is because rising national incomes provide the resources to make sustained investments in health, education, and infrastructure, while rising household incomes (along with female education) also improve food security and reduce fertility rates. There are potentially strong synergies between nutrition-specific and nutrition- sensitive interventions, including education and training programs and general investments in women's education. Effective policies to fight childhood undernourishment will therefore be built upon multisectoral programs that contain both of these components.

References

Heltberg, R. 2009. "Malnutrition, Poverty, and Economic Growth." *Health Economics* 18 (1): 77–88.

Smith, L. C., and L. Haddad. 2000. *Explaining Child Malnutrition in Developing Countries: A Cross-Country Analysis.* Washington, DC: International Food Policy Research Institute.

Webb, P., and S. A. Block. 2010. "Support for Agriculture during Economic Transformation: Impacts on Poverty and Undernutrition." *Proceedings of the National Academy of Sciences of the United States of America,* December 20.

Chapter 6

Growth Is Good, but Is Not Enough to Improve Nutrition

Olivier Ecker, Clemens Breisinger, and Karl Pauw

While it is generally agreed that growth is a necessary precondition for reducing poverty, relatively little is known about the relationship between economic growth and nutrition and, hence, how economic policies can be leveraged to improve nutrition. This chapter argues that growth is good, but is not enough to improve nutrition. During the early stages of development, growth helps reduce the prevalence of calorie deficiency, and, in most countries, agricultural growth plays a key role. But malnutrition becomes less responsive to growth as its prevalence rate declines, so economic diversification into the manufacturing and service sectors becomes necessary to leverage further reductions in malnutrition, especially as people migrate into urban areas. Nevertheless, growth—whether driven by the agriculture or nonagriculture sectors—is insufficient to address child malnutrition and reduce micronutrient malnutrition in all their dimensions. Strategic investments and special programs are needed in the complementary sectors of health and education as well.

These findings are based on cross-country analyses that explore the general relationship between growth and malnutrition in the process of development. To complement these findings, forward-looking economic modeling applied to an agriculture-based economy (Malawi) and an oil-based economy (Yemen) assess the impacts of alternative policies on growth and nutrition outcomes. The conceptual framework underlying the country-specific economic analyses is displayed in Box 1.

Cross-Country Analyses

Growth is good for nutrition, but the plotted graphs in Figures 1 and 2 show that some countries significantly deviate from the general growth–nutrition path. While some countries have been successful in leveraging growth for improved nutrition outcomes others have seen nutrition actually deteriorate despite growth. So, in what

This chapter is based on the authors' 2020 Conference Paper, *Growth Is Good, but Is Not Enough to Improve Nutrition* (Washington, DC: International Food Policy Research Institute, 2011).

Box 1   Methodology and Conceptual Framework

By combining macroeconomic factors with sector and household issues, the new conceptual framework underlying this chapter expands on the common perspective of food security as primarily a household-level problem. It explicitly accounts for the role of sectors that are most relevant to improving people's nutritional status: agriculture, trade and infrastructure, and health and education. In this way, the framework emphasizes the need for an integrated, cross-sector approach to improving nutrition, and includes the major pathways through which policies and external shocks (such as food price crises) translate into nutrition outcomes. This framework is applied by linking economywide, dynamic computable general equilibrium models with household and child nutrition simulation models to enable the effects of sector-level economic growth and policies affecting people's nutritional status to be estimated consistently. The resulting findings offer evidence of the potential impacts of policies under different conditions, ultimately having implications for policy choices and priorities.

FIGur E 1   Relationship between undernourishment and GDP

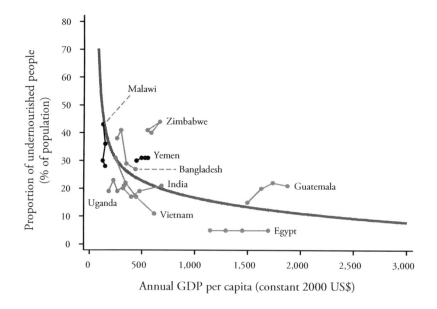

Source: Ecker, Breisinger, and Pauw 2011.

FIGur E 2 Relationship between child malnutrition and GDP

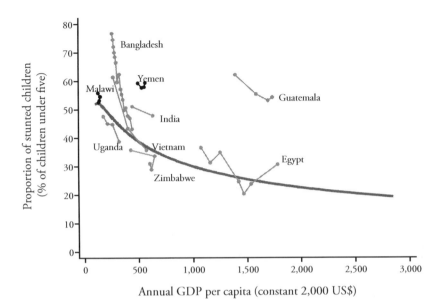

Source: Ecker, Breisinger, and Pauw 2011.

way and to what extent does growth contribute to nutrition outcomes, and how can policies be designed to better leverage growth for nutrition improvements? To answer these questions, the authors conducted two country case studies.

Complementary Case Studies: Malawi and Yemen

Malawi and Yemen are both low-income countries with high levels of malnutrition. Malawi's economy is agriculture-based and features limited economic diversity whereas Yemen has an oil-based economy and a relatively small agriculture sector. The nature of the nutrition challenge in the two countries is also inherently different. In Malawi, micronutrient deficiencies—especially in iron, zinc, vitamin A, and folate—are of particular concern; in Yemen, child malnutrition is extremely widespread in alarmingly severe forms. By capturing a broad range of nutritional challenges, these case studies illustrate country-specific issues while simultaneously providing important general policy lessons on the linkages between agricultural and nonagricultural growth and nutrition outcomes, especially for countries in Africa and the Middle East.

For each of the case studies, three different policy scenarios were explored. For Yemen, the three scenarios, simulated for 2010–20, are (1) a baseline scenario reflecting the growth patterns of the recent past; (2) an agricultural reform scenario under which reform aims to accelerate agricultural growth and increase agricultural output for rural income generation, thereby improving food security; and (3) a promising sector growth path that promotes growth in the manufacturing and service sectors (see Table 1).

For Malawi, the period of high agricultural growth experienced between 2005 and 2010—due almost entirely to rapid maize yield improvements under the Farm Input Subsidy Program (FISP)—was replicated. For the forward-looking period (2010–20), two further scenarios are modeled, namely (1) a return to the more moderate long-term growth rate experienced prior to the introduction of FISP, a scenario based on the assumption that Malawi will not be able to maintain the maize-led growth momentum generated under FISP; and (2) a broad-based agricultural growth path in which it is assumed that Malawi maintains its growth momentum through rapid diversification of the agriculture sector under the Agricultural Sector-Wide Approach currently being implemented (see Table 2).

TABl E 1 S   ummary of policy scenarios, Yemen case study

Yemen	1. Baseline scenario			2. agricultural policy reform			3. Promising sector growth		
	2009	2015	2020	2009	2015	2020	2009	2015	2020
Growth (%)									
National GDP	6.6	3.9	3.6	6.6	4.8	4.4	6.6	7.1	7.0
Agriculture	5.1	2.6	2.1	5.1	4.1	4.3	5.1	3.5	2.8
Industry	11.2	6.4	4.5	11.2	7.7	5.6	11.2	10.7	9.3
Services	6.3	5.1	4.7	6.3	6.0	5.4	6.3	8.8	8.0
Malnutrition									
Proportion of calorie-deficient people (%)	32.1	25.3	24.3	32.1	24.1	21.9	32.1	20.4	15.2
Rural	37.3	31.0	29.7	37.3	29.4	26.6	37.3	24.9	18.5
Farm	33.4	26.7	25.4	33.4	23.2	18.8	33.4	21.0	14.0
Nonfarm	39.2	33.0	31.8	39.2	32.4	30.3	39.2	26.8	20.7
Urban	17.8	9.7	9.3	17.8	9.4	8.9	17.8	7.8	6.1
No. of calorie-deficient people (millions)	7.48	7.04	7.83	7.48		6.70	7.48	5.67	4.90
Proportion of stunted children under five (%)	59.4	58.1	57.8	59.4	57.9	57.5	59.4	57.0	55.3
Rural	63.4	62.3	61.9	63.4	61.9	61.6	63.4	61.2	59.7
Urban	47.9	46.3	46.0	47.9	46.1	45.6	47.9	44.7	42.5

Source: Constructed by authors.

TABl E 2 S   ummary of policy scenarios, Malawi case study

Malawi	1. Past maize-led growth path		2. Return to long-term growth		3. Broad-based agricultural growth	
	2004	2010	2015	2020	2015	2020
Growth (%)						
National GDP	6.8	5.9	4.0	4.1	6.4	6.0
Agriculture	8.5	6.0	3.3	3.4	6.5	5.1
Cereals	17.3	8.3	3.0	3.0	8.9	4.4
Export crops	4.9	5.5	4.1	4.0	5.2	7.7
Mining and industry	5.4	5.5	4.6	4.5	6.2	6.8
Construction and services	5.7	5.9	4.6	4.6	6.3	6.8
Malnutrition						
Proportion of deficient people (%)						
Calories	34.8	17.1	10.3	5.9	8.1	3.5
Iron	47.1	27.0	17.1	10.8	14.3	6.6
Zinc	54.5	32.8	20.8	12.9	16.9	7.9
Vitamin A	65.6	56.5	50.6	44.8	48.0	39.5
Folate	37.3	22.7	16.0	10.4	13.4	6.5
No. of deficient people (millions)						
Calories	4.46	2.67	1.88	1.27	1.48	0.74
Iron	6.04	4.21	3.13	2.32	2.62	1.42
Zinc	6.99	5.11	3.81	2.78	3.09	1.71
Vitamin A	8.41	8.81	9.26	9.63	8.79	8.49
Folate	4.79	3.54	2.93	2.23	2.46	1.39

Source: Constructed by authors.

r esults and Associated Policy Implications

The cross-country analyses revealed four major findings. First, growth is of primary importance in reducing undernourishment. Second, the nutritional impact of growth declines as the development process evolves. Third, especially at early stages of a country's development, agricultural growth is critical for reducing undernourishment, indicating that the structure of growth matters for nutrition outcomes. Fourth, malnutrition among young children—an important dimension of overall nutrition—seems to be highly unresponsive to economic growth, which indicates an important difference from the relationship between growth and poverty.

The case studies confirm that growth leads to significantly reduced calorie deficiency in general. In Yemen, under both the agricultural reform scenario, and the promising sector growth scenario the prevalence of calorie deficiency falls below baseline levels, with the result that the number of calorie-deficient people in 2020 will be lower than that of 2009. In Malawi, even a return to the long-term growth trends in 2010–20 leads to further declines in calorie deficiency.

Depending on the country's economic structure and characteristics of its malnourished people, agricultural or nonagricultural growth can be better for improving nutrition. In Malawi, agriculture has a strong potential to contribute to the reduction of malnutrition. This outcome holds for most agriculture-based economies, where agriculture contributes a main share to the national income, and the majority of poor people derive their living from farming. Under these circumstances, nutrition outcomes improve not only among rural households, but also among urban ones, mainly through reduced food prices and economic linkage effects (both of which increase real incomes). In Yemen, growth led by the industry and service sectors is more beneficial for improving nutrition outcomes than agriculture growth. The effects of agriculture growth on malnutrition are limited in Yemen because the majority of the population draws its income from nonagricultural activities, and farmers are not the most malnourished population group. In addition, most foods—especially staples—are imported, so the net consumer benefit accruing from the local price effect of agricultural productivity growth is low.

The role of growth in improving nutrition shifts during the development process. Comparisons between the broad-based agricultural growth and baseline scenarios in the Malawi study reveal that calorie and micronutrient deficiencies become less responsive to growth as prevalence rates decline, at which time economic diversification is needed to leverage further reductions. Thus, this result supports and extends the finding from the Yemen study indicating that the structure of growth across the whole economy and within the sectors is important for improving people's nutritional status in terms of calories and micronutrients (see Box 2).

Neither agricultural growth nor nonagricultural growth is sufficient to improve child nutrition and reduce micronutrient malnutrition as a whole. Results from the country analyses indicate that cross-country differences are more pronounced for the relationships between growth and child malnutrition than they are for the relationships between growth and undernourishment. For example, despite relatively low growth, Bangladesh has achieved impressive results in consistently reducing child malnutrition over time. In contrast, Egypt has experienced relatively high and steady growth over the past three decades with a low rate of poverty and undernourishment, but the prevalence of child malnutrition is largely unrelated and even returned to its early 1990s levels in recent years. Child malnutrition is less responsive to both overall growth and agricultural growth throughout the process of economic development, so that non-income related factors (such as information and knowledge) and individual health and healthcare seem to matter more in reducing child malnutrition than in reducing undernourishment, especially at later stages of development. This general finding is also confirmed by the results of the case studies. Even with decisive policy reform in Yemen resulting in rapid growth acceleration, child malnutrition remains at unacceptably high levels. In addition, despite reduced deficiencies in calories, iron, zinc, and folate, vitamin-A deficiency in Malawi remains largely unresponsive to economic growth. Although the proportion of people with a vitamin-A deficiency declined due to Malawi's rapidly growing population, the actual number of deficient people increased.

Box 2   the importance of n on-income Measures in e valuating Development Outcomes

In highlighting the absence of links between growth and certain dimensions of nutrition, the results of this study strongly support the use of non-income measurements (for example, nutrition and health status) to complement income-based measurements (for example, poverty) in evaluating develop-ment outcomes. The concepts of being "well-nourished" or "malnourished" are intuitive, and nutrition impacts can be more directly measured through anthropometric indicators. These indicators are typically provided for young children—the most vulnerable population group—and therefore consider distributional issues; they are not subject to arbitrary assumptions about costs and individual needs. An even stronger argument for advancing the role of nutrition in the development agenda is that malnutrition lowers productiv-ity and has serious long-term consequences for development by limiting the physical and mental potential of people—particularly children—thereby limiting the development potential of future generations.

Consequently, policy reform supporting both agricultural and nonagricultural growth needs to be accompanied by strategic investments and targeted programs to tackle child malnutrition. Globally, persistent and widespread child malnutri-tion and the low responsiveness of child nutrition to economic development are particularly alarming. Necessary actions include: (1) investments in infrastructure (especially to expand drinking-water networks), health, and education; (2) programs to improve child and maternal nutrition and health (for example, through birthing assistance and pre- and post-natal care); (3) education campaigns on child feeding practices (including breastfeeding), appropriate diets, proper hygiene, and disease and illness prevention and treatment; (4) child growth monitoring; (5) immuniza-tion campaigns; and (6) nutrient-supplementation programs. Actions to promote gender equality, women's empowerment, and family planning should also be taken. While the evidence shows that proposed investments and programs have high rates of return in the vast majority of cases, they require political will and financial resources, reinforcing the importance of increased revenues from growth.

Specific investments and programs are also needed to effectively reduce micro-nutrient malnutrition. Calorie deficiency and some micronutrient deficiencies decline in the process of economic development, but other micronutrient deficien-cies are less responsive to growing incomes. Possible avenues for directly reducing these deficiencies are programs that distribute nutrient supplements to the most deficient people, mass fortification of commonly consumed foods and condiments, and biofortification. More research investments are clearly needed to enable further exploration and utilization of the potentials of biofortification. Nonetheless, addressing the causes of micronutrient malnutrition inevitably requires programs that support dietary diversification by providing education on nutritious, well-balanced diets. Without this understanding, the nutritional impact of interventions that increase people's economic access to improved nutrition will be strictly limited. Measures that enhance people's direct access to fruits, vegetables, and animal products include programs promoting home and school gardens, small-scale livestock husbandry, and aquaculture. Investments in programs that improve people's health and hygiene are also necessary to reduce secondary malnutrition, which causes nutritional deficiencies through infection, illness, and disease.

Chapter 7

The Role of Agricultural Growth in Reducing Poverty and Hunger: The Case of Tanzania

Karl Pauw and James Thurlow

I n recent times, many countries, particularly in Sub-Saharan Africa and Southeast Asia, have been left puzzled by their failure to improve nutritional outcomes despite prolonged periods of rapid economic growth, in some cases accompanied by rising incomes among the poor. The Tanzanian economy is one example of a country that failed to reap the benefits of sustained rapid growth. National gross domestic product (GDP) grew at 6.6 percent per year during 1998–2007, while agricultural growth, often regarded as instrumental in lowering poverty rates in agrarian-based developing countries, averaged a respectable 4.4 percent during the period (MOFEA 2008). Yet, between 2001 and 2007, Tanzania's poverty rate only fell from 35.7 to 33.6 percent, while the share of the population consuming insufficient calories declined marginally from 25.0 to 23.6 percent (NBS 2010).

This raises questions about the nature of the interrelationships among economic growth, poverty, and nutrition, and more specifically, how the *structure* of growth matters for poverty and nutrition. With respect to the latter, a particularly important question in agrarian-based developing countries, such as Tanzania, is how *agricultural growth* contributes to overall economic growth, poverty, and nutrition. To address these questions, an economywide model of Tanzania is linked with microlevel poverty and nutrition models to (1) show how the current structure of growth resulted in the weak poverty and nutrition outcomes and (2) examine how accelerated, broad-based agricultural growth can contribute to higher overall growth and more rapid reductions in income poverty and hunger. Finally, this chapter examines more closely the growth, poverty, and nutrition contributions of agricultural subsectors in order to identify priority sectors. (See Box 1 for information on the study's design.)

This chapter is based on the authors' IFPRI Discussion Paper (947), *Agricultural Growth, Poverty, and Nutrition in Tanzania* (Washington, DC: International Food Policy Research Institute, 2010).

Box 1   Methodology and Conceptual Framework

Several studies highlight economic growth's sectoral structure as a key determinant of income distribution changes, and also of the strength of the growth–poverty relationship (Ravallion and Datt 1996; Mellor 1999; Diao, Hazell, and Thurlow 2010). The link between growth and nutrition (or food security), however, is less clear (Timmer 2000). Food security includes three dimensions: availability of sufficient quantities of domestically produced or imported food; access to sufficient resources to acquire a nutritious diet; and utilization of food through adequate diet, water, sanitation, and healthcare. Conceptually, the link between growth and food security resembles that between growth and poverty, at least in terms of the access dimension: economic growth raises disposable incomes and thus consumers' ability to purchase more or better-quality food. However, a comprehensive analysis of growth and food security should also consider how growth impacts the availability and utilization dimensions.

This study attempts to offer the comprehensive analysis needed to truly understand and interpret Tanzania's economic growth by using the Tanzanian recursive-dynamic computable general equilibrium (CGE) model, which is highly disaggregated across economic sectors, commodities, and households (Pauw and Thurlow 2011). Of the 58 commodities in the model, about half are agricultural commodities or processed foods from which households derive nutrients. The 110 household groups in the model explicitly link to economic sectors via factor markets, and hence the CGE model provides a mechanism for understanding how different growth paths (such as agriculture-led versus manufacturing-led growth) affect the level and distribution of household incomes. This is crucial for understanding how growth impacts income poverty and households' access to food.

A general equilibrium framework incorporates both commodity demand and supply, with the latter made up of domestically produced and imported goods. This means the model is useful for considering the availability and access dimensions of food security. Prices are furthermore treated as endogenous in such models, which is important from a consumption modeling perspective. Consumption behavior is modeled on the basis of income and price elasticities estimated for each household group and commodity type. Both poverty and nutrition are affected by changes in income and relative prices. An analysis of nutrition impacts, however, also requires a more in-depth look at relative food price movements. If, for example, the price of calorie-rich maize increases and that of protein-rich meat declines such that the overall food price index does not change, the calorie deficiency rate might decline and the protein deficiency rate might increase, even though the poverty rate remains unchanged. The rich (food) commodity–household specification in the CGE model is useful in this regard, as it captures important differences in consumer spending preferences and responsiveness to income and relative price changes across household types.

Examining Tanzania's Recent Agricultural Performance

An examination of recent production trends suggests that although the agricultural sector in Tanzania as a whole grew rapidly during 1998–2007 (at 4.4 percent per year), growth has been volatile, and the source of this growth has been concentrated among a few crops. Rice and wheat, for example, dominate production trends for cereals, while cotton, tobacco, and sugar production grew almost 10 percent per year. Larger-scale commercial farmers grow these well-performing crops on farms heavily concentrated in the northern and eastern periphery of the country. In contrast, yield for maize, the dominant staple food crop grown extensively by subsistence farmers, remained low due to primitive farming methods. The net effect is that Tanzania, despite favorable agroecological conditions, still relies on imported cereals to meet growing consumer demand.

Root crops, which mainly comprise cassava and potatoes, performed relatively well, growing at more than 4 percent per year. Around 15 percent of harvested land is allocated to root crops, making this subsector one of the drivers of recent agricultural growth. By contrast, pulses, oilseeds and horticultural crops, which are generally regarded as higher-value food crops, performed poorly.

Pulses production declined by more than 4 percent annually, with losses only partially offset by a 5 percent growth in the smaller oilseeds subsector. Vegetable and plantain output also stagnated. Among the noncereal food crops, only fruits performed well, growing at 12 percent per year, although fruit production is concentrated in the northern and eastern regions of Tanzania. Noncereals production has therefore been characterized by slow growth in widely produced crops, and fast growth only in regionally concentrated crops.

Export-oriented crops, such as cotton, sugarcane, and tobacco had some of the fastest growth rates during 2000–07 , expanding at around 10 percent per year and accounting for 17.4 percent of merchandise exports in 2007. However, these crops are also highly concentrated in specific regions. Four-fifths of cotton and tobacco, both important smallholder crops, is grown only in specific regions (for example, cotton in the western and lake regions and tobacco in the western and highlands regions). Similarly, around four-fifths of sugarcane is grown in the eastern and northern regions, although sugarcane is mostly grown on larger-scale farms. Coffee and cashew nuts are also important export crops, but their production has declined in recent years.

Tanzania's aggregate agricultural sector's substantial expansion in recent years suggests broad-based agricultural growth. However, a closer examination of agricultural production data suggests the opposite: the strong performance of a few regionally concentrated crops has driven growth in export agriculture.

Comparing Business-as-Usual Growth to Broad-Based Agricultural Growth

To better understand the poverty and nutritional implications of Tanzania's historical growth path, the CGE model is used to produce a baseline scenario that assumes recent production trends continue during the period 2007–15. This chapter compares these results to a hypothetical scenario with accelerated agricultural growth ("agriculture scenario") in which agricultural GDP growth averages 5.3 percent. This scenario assumes a more broad-based agricultural growth path, with yields for crops that have performed well in the past (such as rice, wheat, and certain export crops) improving only marginally, while poor-performing crops (such as maize, pulses, and vegetables) experience larger yield gains, reflecting their greater growth potential.

The effectiveness of growth achieved under the two scenarios is measured with the aid of two types of elasticity: the poverty-growth elasticity (PGE) and the undernutrition-growth elasticity (UGE). The PGE is the percentage decline in poverty caused by a 1 percent increase in per capita GDP. Similarly, the UGE is the percentage change in the undernutrition rate (or calorie deficiency rate) divided by the percentage change in per capita GDP. Table 1 reports the PGE and UGE results from the baseline and agriculture scenarios. Average annual per capita GDP grew by 3.58 in the baseline scenario and 4.09 percent in the agriculture scenario, while poverty declined by 3.68 and 5.39 percent, respectively. This suggests a PGE of –1.03 in the baseline scenario. In the agriculture scenario, the PGE increases to –1.32. The nutrition module, in turn, shows 3.54 and 4.84 percent declines in the undernutrition rate in the two scenarios. This yields a baseline UGE of –0.99, while in the agriculture scenario, the UGE improves significantly to –1.57.

The results confirm that broad-based agricultural growth greatly strengthens growth's impact on poverty. The UGE also rises substantially under the broad-based agricultural growth scenario, which is a reflection of the increased production and consumption of calorie-rich maize, sorghum, millet, and pulses.

TABLE 1 Modeled poverty- and undernutrition-growth elasticities for Tanzania, 2007–15

	Initial deprivation rate (%)	Final deprivation rate (%)	avg. annual % change in deprivation rate (a)	annual per capita gdP growth (%) (b)	deprivation-growth elasticity (a)/(b)
Baseline scenario					
Poverty rate	40.0	29.6	−3.7	3.6	−1.03
Undernutrition rate	23.5	17.6	−3.5	3.6	−0.99
agriculture scenario					
Poverty rate	40.0	25.7	−5.4	4.1	−1.32
Undernutrition rate	23.5	13.8	−4.8	4.1	−1.57

Source: Pauw and Thurlow 2011.

Identifying Priority Sectors for Agricultural Growth

While the previous section illustrated the benefits of broad-based agricultural growth, ascertaining whether certain agricultural subsectors are more effective than others in improving the poverty and nutritional outcomes of agricultural growth requires further modeling. The structure of growth determines development outcomes in several possible ways. First, poorer households may be more intensively engaged in the production of certain crops or agricultural products. Similarly, some subsectors produce products that poorer households consume more intensively. Growth or price fluctuations in these sectors will therefore have a greater impact on poverty than growth or price fluctuations in other sectors. Second, some agricultural subsectors produce low-cost sources of calories often consumed intensively by nutrient-deficient households, meaning growth and price changes within these sectors may have important nutritional effects. A third factor concerns the level of growth itself, and the fact that some sectors—due to their initial size in the economy, downstream production linkages (such as their production multiplier effects), or growth potential (signified by current yield gaps)—can have a greater impact on overall growth. These three criteria are taken into account when identifying subsectors most effective at reducing poverty and undernutrition in Tanzania.

Comparative results are presented in Table 2. The simulated growth in each subsector achieves the same target agricultural GDP by 2015 in each simulation, thus ensuring that the poverty– and calorie–growth elasticities are directly comparable across subsectors. The three highest poverty–growth elasticities are for growth led by maize, root crops, and pulses and oilseeds. These crops are important expenditure items for households just below the poverty line and are grown more intensively by poorer farm households. In contrast, the poverty–growth elasticity for rice– and wheat–led growth is lower, mainly because these crops are grown in less poor regions of the country and, in the case of wheat, by larger-scale farmers who are less likely to be poor. The calorie–growth elasticities indicate that maize, sorghum and millet, and root crops raise household caloric availability per unit of growth most effectively. Although pulses and oilseeds have high calorie contents, the poor consume these less intensively since the crops are fairly expensive sources of calories. Livestock products have the lowest elasticity—in spite of the relatively high calorie content of meat products—because they are an expensive source of calories and calorie-deficient households consume them less intensively (see Box 2).

Production multipliers provide a useful indicator of the growth linkages of different subsectors. Multiplying each sector's production multiplier by its initial share in agricultural GDP constructs a simple index of the contribution each unit of additional growth within a sector makes to overall GDP. This index, shown in the last column of Table 2, identifies horticulture, livestock, and maize as sectors with the greatest potential to have a meaningful effect on national GDP in Tanzania within the eight-year timeframe of our simulation analysis.

Policy Implications

The analysis here suggests Tanzania's low PGE and UGE result from the current structure of agricultural growth, which favors larger-scale production of rice, wheat, and traditional export crops in specific geographic locations. More rapid growth across a wider range of agricultural subsectors—particularly those that provide

TABLE 2   Poverty, nutrition, and growth effects of agricultural subsector growth, 2007–15

	Poverty-growth elasticity	undernutrition-growth elasticity	size and linkage effects
Maize-led growth	−1.174	−1.477	0.152
Sorghum & millet–led growth	−1.136	−1.348	0.033
Rice & wheat–led growth	−1.100	−1.147	0.106
Root crops–led growth	−1.182	−1.350	0.106
Pulses & oilseeds–led growth	−1.141	−1.161	0.101
Horticulture-led growth	−1.118	−1.092	0.186
Export crops–led growth	−1.096	−1.057	0.098
Livestock-led growth	−1.075	−0.977	0.204

Source: Pauw and Thurlow 2011.

Box 2 g etting the Most Calories for the Money

To avoid the feeling of hunger, poorer consumers often allocate a larger share of their income to food types with high calorie contents and lower costs per calorie. The following table compares the calorie content of different foods in Tanzania, shows how the price per 100 kilocalories (kcal) varies by product, and shows average calories available from different food products for poor and nonpoor households. Livestock products have a higher average calorie content per 100-gram serving compared to most other food types, but they also have a higher price that makes them an expensive energy source. Cereals offer a similar amount of calories per serving, but cost considerably less than livestock.

	average calories per standard serving (*)	Mean price (Tsh) per 100 kcal (†)	average per capita caloric availability		
			Poor (‡)	nonpoor	all
Cereals	294	6.3	1,390	1,885	1,687
Root crops	178	5.5	424	423	423
Pulses & oilseeds	443	10.9	196	411	325
Horticulture	49	19.8	106	240	186
Livestock & processed meat	266	26.0	125	318	241
Sugar & other foods	181	23.5	50	78	27

Source: Authors' calculations using expenditure estimates from HBS 2000/01 and calorie content tables in Lukmanji et al. 2008.

Notes: Kcal = kilocalories; TSh = Tanzanian shilling

* No consumption weights were applied in calculating average calories per food group.

† Mean price is the total expenditure divided by total calorie content per food item.

‡ Poverty line is the 40th percentile of per capita expenditure.

employment to many poor households or that supply goods consumed intensively by undernourished households—will make growth more effective at reducing poverty and undernutrition. It is not only (rural) farm households that benefit from broad-based agricultural growth; (urban) nonfarm households also benefit from lower food prices because lower prices increase disposable income and permit reallocation of spending to food items.

The staple maize, already grown extensively by subsistence smallholders in Tanzania, has important size and growth linkages in the economy in addition to having large PGEs and UGEs. The analysis therefore identifies maize as a priority sector for achieving growth, poverty, and nutrition objectives.

The modeling analysis in this chapter did not explicitly consider how increased agricultural productivity might be achieved or the possible costs of investments, extension services, or subsidies. However, studies for Tanzania and elsewhere routinely highlight locally driven agricultural research (for example, in improved seed varieties or farming methods), rural infrastructure investments, and effective provision of relevant extension services as important ways to raise agricultural productivity (Sanchez, Denning, and Nziguheba 2009; Fan, Nyanga, and Rao 2005; Kilima et al. 2008; Nkonya, Schroeder, and Norman 1997; Thirtle, Lin, and Piesse 2003). Although historically the Tanzanian government has neglected agricultural investments, current development plans indicate a reprioritization of agriculture as a driver of economic growth and socioeconomic development. The results in this chapter provide some indication of which agricultural sectors the government's development plans should prioritize to maximize national growth, poverty, and nutrition outcomes.

References

Diao, X., P. Hazell, and J. Thurlow. 2010. "The Role of Agriculture in African Development." *World Development* 38 (10): 1375–1383.

Fan, S., D. Nyanga, and N. Rao. 2005. *Public Investment and Poverty Reduction in Tanzania.* Development Strategy and Governance Discussion Paper 18. Washington, DC: International Food Policy Research Institute.

Kilima, F. T. M., C. Chung, P. Kenkel, and E. R. Mbiha. 2008. "Impact of Market Reform on Spatial Volatility of Maize Prices in Tanzania." *Journal of Agricultural Economics* 59 (2): 257–270.

Lukmanji, Z., E. Hertzmark, N. Mlingi, V. Assey, G. Ndossi, and W. Fawzi. 2008. *Tanzania Food Composition Tables, First Edition.* Dar es Salaam, Tanzania, and Boston, MA: Muhimbili University of Health and Allied Sciences, Tanzania Food and Nutrition Centre, and Harvard School of Public Health.

Mellor, J. W. 1999. *Faster, More Equitable Growth: The Relation Between Growth in Agriculture and Poverty Reduction.* Cambridge, MA: Harvard University Press.

MOFEA (Ministry of Finance and Economic Afffairs), 2008. *The Economic Survey 2007.* Dar es Salaam, Tanzania.

NBS (National Bureau of Statistics), 2002. *Tanzania: Household Budget Survey 2000/01.* Dar es Salaam, Tanzania.

————, 2010. *Tanzania: Household Budget Survey 2007.* Dar es Salaam, Tanzania.

Pauw, K., and J. Thurlow. 2011. "Agricultural Growth, Poverty, and Nutrition in Tanzania." *Food Policy* 36: 795–804.

Nkonya, E., T. Schroeder, and D. Norman. 1997. "Factors Affecting Adoption of Improved Maize Seed and Fertilizer in Northern Tanzania." *Journal of Agricultural Economics* 48 (1): 1–12.

Ravallion, M., and G. Datt. 1996. "How Important to India's Poor Is the Sectoral Composition of Economic Growth?" *World Bank Economic Review* 10 (1): 1–26.

Sanchez, P. A., G. L. Denning, and G. Nziguheba. 2009. "The African Green Revolution Moves Forward." *Food Security* 1: 37–44.

Thirtle, C., L. Lin, and J. Piesse. 2003. "The Impact of Research-Led Agricultural Productivity Growth on Poverty Reduction in Africa, Asia and Latin America." *World Development* 31 (12): 1959–1975.

Timmer, C. P. 2000. "The Macro Dimensions of Food Security: Economic Growth, Equitable Distribution, and Food Price Stability." *Food Policy* 25: 283–295.

Chapter 8

Feeding the Future's Changing Diets: Implications for Agriculture Markets, Nutrition, and Policy

Siwa Msangi and Mark W. Rosegrant

Setting the Stage

Rising incomes and rapid urbanization in developing countries, particularly in Asia, are creating changes in the composition of global food demand. With increasing incomes, direct per capita food consumption is shifting from maize and coarse grains to wheat and rice. As incomes continue to rise and urbanization continues, a secondary shift from rice to wheat takes place, as seen in East and South Asia.

Income growth in developing countries is driving strong growth in per capita and total meat consumption, leading to strong growth in the feed consumption of cereals, particularly maize. In developed countries, on the other hand, growth in per capita meat and cereal consumption has slowed dramatically as these countries have already reached very high levels of meat consumption in past decades. Food consumption growth (and related animal-feed requirements) largely determine the pace at which supply growth must evolve to keep up with domestic and international demand for agricultural goods. Little research has been conducted on the impact of changing consumption patterns over time on the future outlook of the world agricultural economy and the implications of these consumption changes on nutrition and food security. This chapter addresses this knowledge gap by looking at the implications of changing food consumption patterns and their effects on market prices, food security, and nutrition. Using a model-based approach to understanding the potential outcomes of less meat-intensive diets and the subsequent shift in markets that might result, informed recommendations for policy interventions and further research can be made.

This chapter is based on the authors' 2020 Conference Paper, *Feeding the Future's Changing Diets: Implications for Agriculture Markets, Nutrition, and Policy* (Washington, DC: International Food Policy Research Institute, 2011).

The Future of Food to 2030

Results from the International Model for Policy Analysis of Agricultural Commodities and Trade (IMPACT) illustrate how socioeconomic and demographic changes play out in the medium- to long-term evolution of food consumption for key commodity groups. IMPACT is a partial equilibrium agricultural model for crop and livestock commodities; it was developed by the International Food Policy Research Institute (IFPRI) to project global food supply, food demand, and food security to the year 2020 and beyond (Rosegrant et al. 2001; Rosegrant, Cai, and Cline 2002). Drawing on the IMPACT results, we can examine an alternative set of scenarios that illustrate the implications of changes toward less meat-intensive diets on market dynamics and nutritional outcomes.

Alternative Diet Scenarios

We look at two alternative scenarios in which the consumption pathway toward key food commodities in the IMPACT baseline case is altered to reflect the evolution toward "low-meat" diets in high-income countries (which, in these scenarios, means all Organisation for Economic Co-operation [OECD] countries and other countries as defined by the World Bank [2007]). In the first scenario variant—low meat (LM)—the per capita intake of red meat (beef and lamb) and white meat (poultry and pork) is decreased by half in high-income countries over the projection period, which reflects a change in consumer preferences toward greener diets with lower environmental impact. The second scenario extends this variant to include Brazil and China (LMBC). In the longer background paper that this chapter is based on, we use cross-section data to discuss how the reduction of meat consumption compares to trends seen across higher-income regions. The scenarios implement the time period for diet adjustments so that changes begin in 2010 and are complete by 2015, outlining a relatively rapid period of transition. While we cannot elaborate on the details of policy mechanisms that would lead the countries' consumers to adopt alternative diets within the space of this short chapter, we highlight the implications of these diet changes in a way that is relevant to policymakers.

With the implementation of the LM scenario, the per capita consumption of high-income countries is halved (relative to the baseline) by 2030, whereas the consumption level in developing countries rises, on average, by more than 7 percent to just above 27 kilograms per capita per year. When we also reduce meat consumption in China and Brazil, the consumption levels for Africa and India each increase by another 46 and 48 percent, respectively, bringing the average per capita value for all developing countries (minus China and Brazil) up by nearly 7 kilograms per capita per year. Table 1 shows the price changes that accompany these shifts in per capita consumption. It also shows strong decreases for the 2030 prices of livestock products—especially when Brazil and China also undergo similar diet changes, which more than doubles the effect. Because the scenarios focused on decreasing meat consumption, livestock commodities show the strongest decrease in prices. Cereal prices (especially coarse grains like maize) also decrease appreciably under both low-meat scenario variants due to the decreased demand for livestock feed that would be expected when herd sizes are reduced in response to lower livestock product prices.

The effect that less demand for meat has on "releasing" grain for food use is accompanied by a small increase in the per capita consumption of cereals under the two low-meat scenarios. There is not much overlap in food and feed uses for coarse grains like sorghum and maize outside of Sub-Saharan Africa and other developing regions, where the strongest increase in per capita cereals consumption for both low-meat variants occurs. This effect would, of course, not apply to commodities like meal byproducts, which are used exclusively for animal feed and drop strongly in price under both low-meat diet scenarios (see Table 1). If the LMBC scenario

TAbl e 1   world prices of key commodities under baseline and alternative diet scenarios for high-income countries (HiC), Brazil, and China (US$/mt)

	2000	2030 baseline	2030 HiC low meat (LM)	% change from baseline in 2030	2030 HiC + Brazil & China low meat (LMBC)	% change from baseline in 2030
beef	1,971	2,041	1,654	−19	1,252	−38
pork	899	857	657	−23	351	−59
lamb/goat	2,831	2,883	2,546	−12	1,911	−33
poultry	1,245	1,189	923	−22	546	−53
eggs	764	722	711	−2	676	−6
milk	308	340	341	0	341	0
rice	208	265	265	0	268	1
wheat	115	138	136	−2	129	−7
maize	89	148	138	−6	121	−18
other coarse grains	68	79	73	−8	63	−20
soybean	203	300	299	0	298	0
potato	213	180	178	−1	176	−2
sweet potato & yam	476	471	455	−3	425	−10
cassava	64	66	64	−2	62	−7
meal	189	373	344	−8	293	−21

Source: IMPACT model projections.

were expanded to more countries, beyond the HIC regions, China, and Brazil, we would expect to see further reductions in prices of grains and meat products, as livestock demand growth slows over time and more cereals are released from feed consumption.

Implications for Nutrition and Food Security

Looking beyond the change in food consumption patterns and commodity price impacts implied by the results, we can also consider the possible implications of changes across the range of food products for food security. Given the previously discussed supply-and-demand patterns, the IMPACT model infers a trend in levels of malnutrition among the vulnerable demographic of children aged zero to five. Malnutrition's determinants are derived primarily from the four indicators first established by Smith and Haddad: per capita calorie availability, access to clean drinking water, rates of secondary schooling for women, and the ratio of female-to-male life expectancy (2000). These determinants are consistent with the four-pillared food security concept underlining the Food and Agriculture Organization of the United Nations' conceptual framework, where availability, along with access utilization and stability, account for food security status among vulnerable populations. IMPACT's methodology for tracking child malnutrition is based on this work, and is implemented through an analytical relationship that is parameterized by the statistical coefficients derived by Smith and Haddad's work.

Our analysis shows changes in per capita calorie availability are consistent with the simulated changes in per capita consumption in both low-meat scenarios (LM and LMBC). All regions saw an increase in per capita availability—save those directly targeted in the scenarios—which reflects the increases in per capita consumption that accompany the decreases in cereal and meat prices on the world market.

Implications for Food Policy

Following the quantitative scheme based on the Smith/Haddad relationship and drawing from the scenario-driven changes in per capita calorie consumption, child malnutrition changes demonstrate the calorie-releasing effect of reducing livestock consumption, production, and feed demand in both low-meat scenario variants (see Table 2).

Under the low-meat scenario that targets only high-income countries, the decrease of child malnutrition in Sub-Saharan Africa is nearly half a million; the inclusion of Brazil and China in the scenario results in an even larger improvement, increasing the magnitude of the reduction of undernourished children to

TAbl e 2 **Child malnutrition under baseline and diet scenarios for high-income countries (HiC), Brazil, and China (millions of children aged 0–5)**

	t otal malnourished children		t otal change in malnourishment from baseline	
	2000	2030 baseline	2030 HiC low meat (LM)	2030 HiC + Brazil & China low meat (LMBC)
Northern SS Africa	11.3	15.6	−0.1	−0.3
Western SS Africa	6.6	10.1	−0.1	−0.3
Eastern SS Africa	3.2	4.6	−0.1	−0.2
Southern SS Africa	4.6	7.4	−0.1	−0.3
All of SS Africa	32.1	44.3	−0.4	−1.3
West Asia and North Africa	6.2	4.3	−0.1	−0.1
South Asia	75.6	62.8	−0.1	−0.4
South Asia minus India	19.2	19.6	0.0	−0.1
Southeast Asia	13.5	11.5	0.0	−0.1
East Asia	10.7	4.9	−0.1	−0.2
All of Asia	99.9	79.2	−0.2	−0.6
All of Latin America	7.7	6.5	−0.1	−0.2
All Developing*	146.5	134.9	−0.7	−2.2

Source: IMPACT model projections.

*Includes China and Brazil.

1.3 million. Child malnutrition also improves in South Asia under both low-meat scenarios, although to a lesser extent (0.1 million fewer undernourished children for the LM case, which increases to 0.4 million fewer when China and Brazil are included). On the whole, the benefits of releasing grains from livestock production systems by reducing the demand for meat has a sizable effect on decreasing malnutrition—especially for those regions that consume coarse grains like maize and sorghum more as food than as feed for livestock (as is the case in Sub-Saharan Africa). It should be noted that IMPACT's partial-equilibrium framework does not capture any changes to farmers' incomes that are caused by these shifts in the supply and revenue generated from crop and livestock products. Another possible poverty-reducing and (ultimately) nutrition-enhancing benefit not captured by this framework is the positive effects of less meat consumption on human health, especially in higher-income countries where a number of chronic diseases can be linked to excesses in dietary intakes.

Since halting or altering urbanization, population growth, and income growth is not a plausible policy instrument for influencing consumption behavior, the only avenue that policy can take is to influence consumers themselves to diversify their diets and move away from a meat-intensive regime. Nutrition education, as part of a long-term health education program that strives to target diverse demographics, could be a useful instrument toward that end. Such a program's influence, however, would only be realized gradually over time, similarly to the patterns seen in other health-oriented education efforts such as AIDS-awareness campaigns.

A more direct means to exert influence would be to promote healthy diets within government-sponsored feeding programs (for example, relief efforts or school lunch programs), although the benefits would be limited to the intervention's target population. While taxes on meat have been proposed as an additional mechanism to encourage consumers to change their eating habits, no effort has been success-ful in richer countries due to inevitable political resistance from powerful interests supporting ranching operations and meat production.

Conclusions

Dietary diversity is a key driver of change in food systems, and it can have a variety of effects on the evolution of food prices, consumption, and other future world food market dynamics. A strong shift toward less-meat-intensive diets significantly decreases the price and consumption of livestock products, as well as cereal com-modities used for animal feed. Reducing high meat consumption in fast-growing countries—like China—has an even bigger impact than reducing meat consump-tion in high-income, OECD countries. If we expanded the scenario with diet change in China and Brazil to include other emerging economies like Indonesia, India, and the faster-growing countries within Latin America and Sub-Saharan Africa, we might see these effects further multiplied. Encouraging diets richer in pulse-based proteins, fruits, and vegetables could have other benefits—aside from just reducing meat consumption—not captured in our analysis. Aside from the obvious nutritional and health benefits, greater consumption of healthier foods in both developed and developing regions could lead to further welfare improve-ments through farmers' additional income earned by supplying fresh horticultural fruits and vegetables to wealthier countries. This is already the case in a number of developing tropical regions.

While diet changes in developed and rapidly growing countries can make a significant impact, this alone cannot bring about long-term improvement of global food security. Instead, significant progress on malnutrition in developing countries will require economic growth that generates employment and reduces inequal-ity and poverty; investments in agricultural and rural development, agricultural research and technologies, and health and education; and the development of infrastructure such as irrigation, domestic water supply, good roads, communications, and effective markets (Rosegrant, Fernandez, and Sinha 2009).

References

Rosegrant, M. W., X. Cai, and S. Cline. 2002. *World Water and Food to 2025: Dealing with Scarcity.* Washington, DC: International Food Policy Research Institute.

Rosegrant, M. W., M. Fernandez, and A. Sinha. 2009. "Looking into the Future for Agriculture and AKST." In *International Assessment of Agricultural Knowledge, Science and Technology for Development (IAASTD) Global Report,* edited by B. D. McIntyre, H. R. Herren, J. Wakhungu, and R. T. Watson. Washington, DC: Island Press, 307–356.

Rosegrant, M. W., M. S. Paisner, S. Meijer, and J. Witcover. 2001. *Global Food Projections to 2020: Emerging Trends and Alternative Futures.* Washington, DC: International Food Policy Research Institute.

Smith, L., and L. Haddad. 2000. *Explaining Child Malnutrition in Developing Countries: A Cross-Country Analysis.* IFPRI Research Report 111. Washington, DC: International Food Policy Research Institute.

World Bank. 2007. *World Development Report 2008: Agriculture for Development.* Washington, DC: International Bank for Reconstruction and Development, World Bank.

Chapter 9

Value Chains for Nutrition

Corinna Hawkes and Marie T. Ruel

Currently, close to 1 billion people suffer from hunger and food insecurity, defined as not having enough calories to live a healthy life. While this number is staggering, the number of people with poor access to nutritious foods rich in essential micronutrients—such as fruits and vegetables, meat, fish, dairy products, and biofortified staple foods—is even more daunting. Deficiencies in micronutrients such as vitamin A, iron, and zinc affect the survival, health, development, and well-being of billions of people; low fruit and vegetable consumption is also associated with increased risk of chronic diseases. Increasing poor people's consumption of nutritious foods is therefore essential to solving malnutrition in all its forms.

Limited availability, economic constraints, lack of knowledge and information, and related lack of demand for nutritious foods are critical factors that limit poor people's access to such foods. In theory, the agriculture sector could help address this problem by helping at-risk groups generate more income and by making nutritious foods more available, affordable, acceptable, and of higher quality. Agriculture-based development programs that aim to improve nutrition have tended to focus on agricultural production and consumption by producer households. Yet the links among what is produced on the farm, the consumer, and the income received by the producer do not stop at the farmgate. Far from it: food is stored, distributed, processed, retailed, prepared, and consumed in a range of ways that affect the availability, affordability, acceptability, and nutritional quality of foods for the consumer. Therefore, if the agriculture sector is to play a more important role in improving nutrition, there needs to be a greater focus on what happens between production and consumption. One way of addressing this issue is to adopt "value-chain" concepts, analysis, and approaches. Value-chain approaches are already used as development strategies to enhance the livelihoods of food producers, but they have, to date, rarely been used explicitly as a tool to achieve nutritional goals, and they have not been sensitive to nutritional concerns. This chapter seeks to identify

This chapter is based on the authors' 2020 Conference Paper, *Value Chains for Nutrition* (Washington, DC: International Food Policy Research Institute, 2011).

if, why, and how value-chain concepts could and should be applied to enhance the ability of agriculture to improve nutrition.

What Are Value Chains, Value-Chain Analysis, and Value-Chain Approaches?

A *value chain* starts with a supply chain: the processes and actors that take a product from its conception to its end use or disposal (see Figure 1). Although a value chain is a form of supply chain, the "value" component imbues it with greater meaning: value is *added* to the product through "value-adding" activities as it passes through the chain. These activities *create* value for the value-chain actors. A value chain can thus be described by what and where value is added in the supply chain for and by these activities and actors. The "value" involved may refer to the value of the product in economic terms, to the value added to the product as it passes through the chain, or to the economic value that is created and captured by the actors in the chain—or to all of these forms of value. "Adding value" may also refer to enhancing the benefit offered by the product relative to its price, as perceived by consumers.

Value-chain analysis involves identifying (1) the actors involved in the chain and the relationship between them; (2) the activities performed by each actor and his or her location; and (3) some form of attribution of value corresponding to the activities and actors in the chain. There are many different ways to conduct value-chain analysis, but all are distinct from other forms of supply-chain analysis by assuming that the value through the chain is affected by the interactions among the different actors and activities, not just the isolated behavior of individual actors in that chain. Value-chain analysis has been used in practice in several areas. For example, private companies use it to enhance competitive strategy, and researchers have used it to examine the processes, causes, and consequences of global industrial integration (globalization).

Value-chain approaches to development have been adopted by several development agencies to encourage greater participation by poor people in modern value chains, including food value chains. These include agricultural value-chain development projects, which tend to focus on some form of "upgrading" as a means of increasing returns to farmers (that is, changing their products, improving their processes, increasing the volume produced, changing their functions, or improving coordination to capture more value).

FiGur e 1 a   simplified representation of a food supply chain

Activities	Actors
Inputs into production	Crop breeders; extension services; seed, agrochemical, and farm machinery companies
Food production	Farmers, agricultural laborers, commodity producers
Primary food storage and processing	Packers, millers, crushers, refiners
Secondary food processing	Processed foods manufacturers, artisan to global
Food distribution, transport, and trade	Importers, exporters brokers, wholesalers
Food retailing and catering	Informal retailers, supermarket chains, restaurants, fast food companies
Food promotion and labeling	Advertising and communications agencies

Food availability — Food affordability — Food acceptability — Food quality

Food consumption and diet quality

Source: Adapted from Hawkes 2009.

Can Adoption of Value-Chain Concepts Help Achieve Nutrition Goals?

The emphasis of value-chain approaches to agricultural development in developing countries so far has been on enhancing the economic benefits of food production (Hawkes and Ruel 2011). In these approaches, consumers have been perceived as the market for farm products, not as actors in the chain whose activities add value to or create value for the product. Yet consumers are actors in food value chains through various activities (such as consumption, lobbying, and so on) and can add value to products from which they perceive enhanced benefits (for example, nutritional value).

Value-chain approaches to agricultural development to date have also tended to perceive value chains as only being responsive to consumers; rarely have they considered the influence the chain has on consumption patterns. Yet in practice, production and consumption are mutually constitutive processes. Consumption influences production—more so since the shift toward a globalized market model. But production also influences consumption—with postproduction activities and actors becoming more important in the globalizing era.

Through their focus on value, value chains provide a theoretical framework that captures these mutually constitutive processes. On the supply side, constructing a value chain enables one to identify where nutritional value can be created, as well as where economic value can be created for the actors in the supply chain. On the demand side, the concept of value can be extended to the consumers' "perception of value." Value-chain approaches can then be applied to enhance the perception of value of nutritious foods while also creating economic benefits for agricultural actors. Thus emerges a reconceptualized theory of "value chains for nutrition," in which consumers become actors rather than just a "market," nutrition and public health goals become paramount in value chain development, and both at-risk producers and consumers are considered.

Adopting value-chain concepts thus has enormous potential to help increase both the supply of nutritious foods to the poor and their demand for those foods (see Box 1). First, value-chain analysis can be used to assess why foods are or are not available in specific communities, why foods cost what they do, how the nutrient quality of foods changes through the chain, and how public interventions and policies—such as providing information and knowledge about the nutritional value of foods or subsidizing or investing in production of nutritious foods (for example vegetables and fruits through public research and development)—can help integrate nutrition into the whole chain. Once problems are identified, value-chain approaches can be used to design and implement solutions to increase the availability, affordability, and quality of nutritious foods. Value-chain analysis can also be used to address acceptability and demand constraints. It can be used, for example, to identify what kind of "value" needs to be added to products to increase consumer acceptability and demand, as well as to determine if adding nutritional value alters the way the consumers "value" the products or their "willingness to pay."

Value-chain concepts can be particularly useful to help achieve these goals because they are concrete and solution oriented while also being expansive in their reach. Since they incorporate all the steps in the chain at all scales in all sectors, value-chain concepts can help identify causes and implement solutions that are not necessarily obvious, or that may even be counterintuitive. Since value-chain concepts explicitly recognize that it is the coordination among the actors that enhances the ability of businesses or sectors to create value, they also encourage the

Box 1   Value Chains for nutrition: examples in action

Value-chain approaches have not to date been applied in the field of nutrition in a consistent or comprehensive way, but there have been some attempts to apply value-chain approaches in a nutrition context (Hawkes and Ruel 2011).

Projects with explicit nutrition goals and related activities:

• *Enhancing the bean value chain in Uganda:* A project to improve bean production, marketing, and consumption as a means of enhancing sustainable livelihoods. In a value-chain framework, actions included research into increasing yields, improving nutrient quality after harvest, understanding consumers' preferences and demand, increasing their awareness of the nutritional and health benefits of beans, and promoting bean consumption (Mazur et al. 2011).

• *Strengthening the value chain for orange-fleshed sweet potato (OFSP) in Mozambique and Uganda:* With the ultimate objective of improving vitamin A intake and status, this project implemented actions at three levels of the value chain—farmers, traders, and consumers. Among many other things, actions included distributing OFSP vines to producers, disseminating results of willingness-to-pay studies to traders, and using mass media and promotional events to raise consumer awareness of the nutritional benefits of OFSP and promote their consumption, especially among nutritionally vulnerable mothers and young children (Coote et al. 2011).

• *Developing nutrition programs in Sierra Leone:* REACH (the Renewed Efforts Against Child Hunger partnership) is currently developing a value-chain framework for programs involving food purchases from local farmers. The aim is to increase the demand for nutritious foods while augmenting the incomes of small farmers (Torgerson et al. in Hawkes and Ruel 2011).

Projects that incorporate nutrition or health concerns but do not have specific nutrition goals:

• *Developing a dairy value chain for smallholders in Zambia:* Land O'Lakes International Development used a market-based, value-chain approach in *its work with small farmers in Zambia.* The objective was to reduce household food insecurity through increased incomes from the sale of milk and other dairy products and increase the demand for dairy products among producers and consumers (Grant and Russell in Hawkes and Ruel 2011).

Program that incorporates value-chain concepts but does not have specific nutrition goals:

• *Creating value for producers in the value chain for ready-to-use therapeutic foods (RUTFs) in Ethiopia:* Hilina, a food-processing company in Ethiopia, worked with local producers to eliminate aflatoxin contamination in peanuts, thereby enabling them to supply ingredients for the production of RUTFs (fortified processed food used to treat severe acute malnutrition). The ultimate objective was to enable the local production and supply of RUTFs at a reduced cost (Jones in Hawkes and Ruel 2011).

type of coordinated, cross-sectoral approaches that are critically needed to address malnutrition. They can provide a framework for coordinating actions and actors and for identifying and engaging the sectors that need to be involved. These tasks are particularly relevant for any effort to coordinate the agricultural and health sectors. Value-chain concepts also provide a framework for measuring some of the trade-offs between economic returns and nutrition benefits from agriculture.

It is also important to recognize, however, that there are some significant potential limitations to applying value-chain concepts to achieve nutrition goals. The focus of value-chain development so far has been on adding value in the chain, often in ways that make products more expensive for consumers. There may be less scope to add value to products that are targeted to poor consumers — for example, undifferentiated commodities, often distributed outside of formal food markets — making these chains an apparently less appropriate target for value-chain development. Value chains also focus on single food commodities, whereas a healthy and high-quality diet consists of a combination of different foods. Finally, value-chain approaches focus on private competitive markets and have given little attention to making nutritious foods available in settings like food aid distribution points or institutional markets like schools, which are potentially important for specific at-risk groups.

Applying Value-Chain Concepts to Achieve Nutrition Goals

The case studies of value chains for nutrition (Box 1) show that there is not just one way to conduct a value-chain analysis, apply a value-chain approach, or examine the implications of an existing value chain. They suggest unifying principles for the application of value-chain concepts that take into account the benefits of applying value-chain concepts, as well as the very real limitations.

1. *Start with explicit nutrition goals.* While there is not a single value-chain-for-nutrition approach, all value-chain approaches to nutrition should focus on a clearly stated, outcome-oriented nutrition goal.

2. *Clearly define the nutrition problem.* Although value chains focus on a single commodity, value-chain approaches can be consistent with total diet or systems-based approaches when an intervention begins by identifying core food and nutrient gaps. Once identified, these gaps—and associated health problems—can be addressed by targeting one or more food value chains.

3. *Create and capture value for nutrition.* Although value-chain approaches to nutrition do need to consider economic value for actors in the chain—a necessary component of any value-chain approach—they should also consider the value for nutrition. The case studies show that increases in economic value for vulnerable value-chain actors can be associated with increased value for nutrition, even if this is not their original intention.

4. *Be expansive in the search for solutions, but tailor them to context.* The search for solutions should take the whole value chain—including different sectors and actors at different scales—into account, but the application of solutions should be tailored to circumstance.

5. *Focus on the coordination of the whole chain.* Improving coordination may involve intervening at several points along the chain or taking a few actions to fix coordination problems or create incentives for change along the chain. Coordination also requires developing alliances between the actors involved.

6. *Add value not only for nutrition but also for actors along the value chain.* Solutions for nutrition that do not work for actors within the value chain are not value-chain solutions. Rather, nutrition-oriented activities should become a solution to the problems faced by these actors as well, thus adding value for both consumers and actors along the value chain.

7. *Take a broader view of adding value for producers and consumers.* Consumers' willingness to pay may actually increase as products offer new attributes (such as greater nutritional value or desirability), even among poor people. There are also ways to add value for producers without making the product less affordable for consumers—for example, value-chain activities may mean that producers are able to produce more to supply a larger market.

8. *Focus on meeting, increasing, and creating demand.* Applying value-chain concepts to nutrition should involve taking a broad approach to demand by including consumers' unmet and uncreated demand, not just existing demand. Poor people, for instance, may have a latent demand for more diverse diets that include a variety of micronutrient-rich foods.

9. *Create a policy environment in which better nutrition is valued.* Developing value chains for nutrition will be successful at a broader scale only if the policy environment creates incentives for the actors in the chain to value nutrition and change their behavior accordingly.

Conclusions

To date, the use of value-chain concepts for nutrition has been minimal; only a few such interventions have occurred, and none of these actually measure nutritional impact. Yet value-chain concepts offer considerable potential for enhancing efforts to improve nutrition, and they provide a framework within which opportunities for leveraging agriculture for nutrition can be identified and implemented. This is especially the case given the current focus on value-chain development for agriculture in international development, which provides an opportunity to build in nutrition concerns.

The nascent field of value chains for nutrition should now focus on diagnosing and implementing interventions, keeping in mind that these interventions cannot be identified ahead of time. Each value-chain problem will require its own set of solutions, which could involve anything from information and education, research and technology, chain reorganization, and new financial incentives to development of new policies and standards. Nonetheless, certain principles should be followed, especially the core value-chain concepts concerning coordination, the consideration of the whole chain, and the attribution of some form of value. All value chains inherently involve economic value—a value chain is not a value chain without this. And enhancing nutrition is part of human and economic welfare. But value chains for nutrition must also identify the value to nutrition as it is added, created, gained, and lost throughout the chain, as a separate, though linked, component. The value to the consumer must also be fully incorporated in its dimensions. It is possible to develop value chains to improve nutrition while also providing solutions to development challenges in other sectors—not least, in agriculture.

re Fer eNCeS

Coote, C., K. Tomlins, J. Massingue, J. Okwadi, and A. Westby. 2011. *Understanding Consumer Decisionmaking to Assist Sustainable Marketing of Vitamin A–Rich Sweet Potato in Mozambique and Uga nda.* 2020 Conference Note 2. Washington, DC: International Food Policy Research Institute.

Hawkes, C. 2009. "Identifying Innovative Interventions to Promote Healthy Eating Using Consumption-Oriented Food Supply Chain Analysis." *Journal of Hunger and Environmental Nutrition* 4 (3 and 4): 336–56.

Hawkes, C., and M. T. Ruel. 2011. *Value Chains for Nutrition.* 2020 Conference Paper. Washington, DC: International Food Policy Research Institute, 2011.

Mazur, R., H. K. Musoke, D. Nakimbugwe, and M. Ugen. 2011. *Enhancing Nutritional Value and Marketability of Beans through Research and Strengthening Key Value Chain Stakeholders in Uganda.* 2020 Conference Note 1. Washington, DC: International Food Policy Research Institute.

Chapter 10

Biofortification: Leveraging Agriculture to Reduce Hidden Hunger

Howarth Bouis and Yassir Islam

Micronutrient Malnutrition: A Hidden Hunger

Experts estimate that 2 billion people, mostly in poorer countries, suffer from micronutrient malnutrition, also known as hidden hunger (WHO and FAO 2006). This is caused by a lack of critical micronutrients such as vitamin A, zinc, and iron in the diet. Hidden hunger impairs the mental and physical development of children and adolescents and can result in lower IQ, stunting, and blindness; women and children are especially vulnerable. Hidden hunger also reduces the productivity of adult men and women due to increased risk of illness and reduced work capacity.

In 2008, the *Lancet* published a landmark series of articles on maternal and child undernutrition highlighting the extent of hidden hunger. One study found that men who had received nutrition supplements (that included micronutrients) from ages 0–36 months earned a higher hourly wage than men who had not received the supplements. The group that received nutrition supplements from ages 0–24 months earned 46 percent higher-than-average wages (Hoddinott et al. 2008). Hidden hunger's enormous consequences, not only to individuals but also to society through reduced economic productivity, have brought more attention to the issue recently. Also in 2008, a panel of noted economists that included five Nobel Laureates, ranked efforts to reduce hidden hunger among the most cost-effective solutions to global challenges. One of these efforts, biofortification, was ranked fifth.[1]

---

1. See Copenhagen Consensus 2008: Results, www.copenhagenconsensus.com/Home.aspx and Copenhagen Consensus, "Micronutrient Fortification and Biofortification," www.copenhagen-consensus.com/Default.aspx?ID=1456

This chapter is based on H. E. Bouis and R. M. Welch, "Biofortification—A Sustainable Agricultural Strategy for Reducing Micronutrient Malnutrition in the Global South," *Crop Science* 50, no. 2 (2010): S1–S13.

Leveraging Agriculture to Improve Nutrition through Biofortification

Agriculture is the primary source of nutrients necessary for a healthy life, but agricultural policies and technologies have focused on improving profitability at the farm and agroindustry levels, not on improving nutrition (Bouis and Welch 2010). Given the prevalence of hidden hunger, there is growing interest in the role agriculture should play in improving nutrition, in particular by paying more attention to the nutritional quality of food.

Biofortification is a scientific method for improving the nutritional value of foods already consumed by those suffering from hidden hunger (Bouis et al. 2011). Scientists first breed crops whose edible portions (seed, tuber, or roots, for example) have higher amounts of nutrients. Malnourished communities receive these biofortified crops to grow and eat. When consumed regularly, biofortified foods can contribute to body stores of micronutrients throughout the life cycle. This strategy should contribute to the overall reduction of micronutrient deficiencies in a population, but it is not expected to *treat* micronutrient deficiencies or eliminate them in all population groups.

The Biofortification Process

Biofortification requires experts from different fields to work together. Plant breeders explore the full spectrum of crop genetic diversity, especially seed banks, to first identify nutrient-rich germplasm, or lines, of food crops that can be used to breed more nutritious varieties. These lines are then crossed with established high-yielding lines to breed new crop varieties that not only have higher amounts of a desired nutrient, but also are high yielding and competitive with other nonbiofortified varieties. Plant breeders can use both conventional plant breeding and transgenic methods to reach their breeding targets. (For a complementary approach to biofortification, see Box 1.)

Nutritionists determine the additional amount of a nutrient a food crop must provide to measurably improve nutrition when that crop is harvested, processed or cooked, and eaten. To do so, nutritionists must account for

- nutrient losses after the crop is harvested (nutrients can degrade substantially during storage, processing, or cooking),

- the amount of the nutrient that the body actually absorbs from the food (bioavailability), and

- the amount of the staple food actually consumed on a daily basis by age and gender.

Box 1 more than one way to Biofortify

Another approach, referred to as agronomic biofortification, seeks to improve the mineral content of food crops through fertilizer applications, which are applied to the soil or directly to the leaves by foliar spray. The HarvestZinc Fertilizer Project has found that foliar application of zinc fertilizers to wheat can significantly increase zinc concentration in the grain. Depending on the extent of zinc deficiency in soils, zinc fertilizers can contribute to better yield of cereal crops. For more information, please see www.harvestzinc.org.

Source: Cakmak 2008.

These data are then used to set breeding targets for specific nutrients. Once these new crop lines have been bred, they are field-tested by a national agricultural system in multiple locations in target regions where the crop will be grown. This ensures the crops perform well and maintain their nutritional profile, which can be affected by the growing environment. The most promising lines are selected for further testing and eventual release as new varieties through public channels, the private sector, or both.

Nutritionists also test promising new lines and varieties prior to release, to ensure they have a measurable positive impact on the micronutrient status of target communities. This is done through controlled human feeding trials called efficacy studies.

Together with nutritionists, economists conduct studies to evaluate the impact of production and consumption of biofortified varieties of crops on various livelihoods and health outcomes. Behavioral-change experts help identify what drives consumption patterns and how biofortified crops and foods can be better promoted. Ultimately, a range of skills in farm extension, seed replication and distribution, and product marketing is also needed to ensure the successful adoption of the final product by both producers and consumers in target communities.

Special consideration should be given to crops whose color or taste is changed by increasing nutrient levels. To date, this has been the case when crops such as sweet potato, cassava, and maize have been enhanced with vitamin A. These crops turn from a typical white or pale yellow to a deeper yellow or orange in color due to the higher levels of beta-carotene (a precursor to vitamin A) they now contain. This orange color can be an asset in branding or can help consumers identify more nutritious varieties.

HarvestPlus, a component of the CGIAR Research Program on Agriculture for Improved Nutrition and Health, leads a global effort to develop and deliver biofortified staple food crops with one or more of three most limiting nutrients in the diets of the poor: vitamin A, zinc, and iron (Brown 1991). HarvestPlus is an interdisciplinary program that works with experts in more than 40 countries. A release schedule for HarvestPlus crops is shown in Table 1. Other global, regional, and country biofortification programs are working around the world.

Advantages of Biofortification

Dietary diversity is the ultimate long-term solution to minimizing hidden hunger. This will require substantial increases in income for the poor so they are able to afford more nutritious nonstaple foods such as vegetables, fruits, and animal products. Biofortification can be effective in reducing hidden hunger as part of a strategy that includes dietary diversification and other interventions such as supplementation and commercial fortification.

Biofortification has four main advantages when applied in the context of the poor in developing countries. First, it targets the poor who eat large amounts of food staples daily. Second, biofortification targets rural areas where it is estimated that 75 percent of the poor live mostly as subsistence or smallholder farmers, or landless laborers. These populations rely largely on cheaper and more widely available

TABLe 1   HarvestPlus target crops and countries

crop	nutrient	target country	traits	release year
Bean	Iron (Zinc)	DR Congo, Rwanda	virus resistance, heat, & drought tolerance	2012
Cassava	Vitamin A	DR Congo, Nigeria	virus resistance	2011
Maize	Vitamin A	Zambia	disease resistance, drought tolerance	2012
Pearl millet	Iron (Zinc)	India	mildew resistance, drought tolerance	2012
Rice	Zinc (Iron)	Bangladesh, India	disease & pest resistance	2013
Sweet potato	Vitamin A	Uganda, Mozambique	virus resistance, drought tolerance	2007
Wheat	Zinc (Iron)	India, Pakistan	disease resistance	2013

Note: HarvestPlus also supports biofortification of the following crops: Banana/Plantain (vitamin A), Lentil (iron, zinc), Potato (iron, zinc), Sorghum (zinc, iron).

Source: HarvestPlus, "Crops," http://www.harvestplus.org/content/crops, accessed January 25, 2011.

staple foods such as rice or maize for sustenance. Despite urbanization and income growth associated with globalization, diets of the rural poor will continue to be heavily based on staple foods like cereals and tuber crops in many regions (Msangi et al. 2010). Expected increases in food prices, exacerbated by climate change, are likely to increase this reliance on staple foods (see Box 2).

Box 2 the challenge of rising food Prices and climate change

Future population and income growth will result in increased demand for food that will outstrip productivity, resulting in higher food prices. Climate change, which adds stress to agricultural systems, has a multiplier effect resulting in even higher food prices. Rising food prices will negatively affect the nutrition of the poor who cope by protecting consumption of staple foods (whose cost has risen) to keep from going hungry. In doing so, they reduce consumption of more expensive nonstaple foods. However, nonstaple foods have higher micronutrient content, so further reducing the already low amounts of these foods that the poor consume will increase micronutrient malnutrition. For example, if poor people in developing countries faced a 50 percent increase in all food prices across the board, and no increase in income, iron intake would fall by 30 percent. In those societies where preference is given to males in the intrahousehold distribution of nonstaple foods, women and children are likely to be most negatively affected. Biofortification can help make up for the expected micronutrient shortfall, especially among poor consumers.

Climate change may also have an impact on the nutritional quality of the crop itself. While rising CO_2 levels may accelerate plant growth initially, some studies suggests that the nutrient content of crops is likely to decline, especially as plants adapt to higher atmospheric CO_2 levels. One review found a decline in micronutrient content. Overall, the evidence on effects of climate change on nutritional quality is mixed and limited. Further research is needed as there is variability in how plants will respond to the different effects of climate change. Biofortification could offer a solution in those instances where crop nutritional quality will decline.

Sources: Bouis, Eozenou, and Rahman 2011; DaMatta et al. 2010; Loladze 2002; and Nelson et al. 2010.

For example, Figure 1 shows the relative share of calories from different types of foods people consume in rural Bangladesh. Staple foods, mostly rice, account for more than 80 percent of the caloric energy intake. Nonstaple plant foods and meat products account for less than 20 percent of energy intake, yet rural Bangladeshis spend almost 60 percent of their food budgets on these more expensive, and more nutritious, foods.

Supplements or fortified food products are often not widely available in rural areas; in fact, coverage of fortified foods in rural areas may be less than one-third.[2] Therefore, locally produced, more nutritious staple food crops could significantly improve nutrition for the rural poor who eat these foods on a daily basis.

Biofortification is cost-effective. After an initial investment in developing bio-fortified crops, those crops can be adapted to various regions at a low additional cost and are available in the food system, year after year. Ex ante research that examined the cost-effectiveness of a variety of staple crops biofortified with provitamin A, iron, and zinc in 12 countries in Africa, Asia, and Latin America found that biofortification could be highly cost-effective, especially in Asia and Africa (Meenakshi 2010). Because this strategy relies on foods people already eat habitually, it is sustainable.

---

2. See Copenhagen Consensus 2008: Results, www. copenhagenconsensus.com/Home.aspx and Copenhagen Consensus, "Micronutrient Fortification and Biofortification," www. copenhagen-consensus.com/Default.aspx?ID=1456.

FIgu Re 1 S   hare of energy source and food budget in rural Bangladesh

Source: HarvestPlus, "Food Crisis," www.harvestplus.org/content/food-crisis.

Seeds, roots, and tubers can usually be saved by farmers and shared with others in their communities. Once the high-nutrition trait is bred into the crops, it is fixed, and the biofortified crops can be grown to deliver better nutrition year after year—without recurring costs.

Biofortification: Limitations and Challenges

Promising as it is, biofortification faces limitations and challenges. First, biofortification requires a paradigm shift. Agricultural science and nutrition are compartmentalized disciplines that must be integrated for biofortification to succeed. Agricultural scientists need to add nutrition objectives to their breeding programs, in addition to standard goals such as productivity and disease resistance. Plant breeders must then work closely with nutritionists to develop breeding targets for nutrients. Nutritionists and health professionals also need to accommodate agriculture-based approaches in their toolbox along with clinical interventions.

Second, biofortification will be widely adopted only when proponents show that these new foods improve nutrition. Most biofortified crops are still in the development pipeline. However, one biofortified staple food crop that has been successfully released is the orange (or orange-fleshed) sweet potato (OSP; see Box 3). As other crops follow, nutritionists will be able to build a body of evidence that biofortification is a viable agriculture-based intervention to improve nutrition.

Third, the amounts of nutrients that can be bred into these crops are generally much lower than can be provided through fortification and supplementation.

Box 3 0   range s weet Potato: a n Emerging s uccess s tory

Varieties of orange sweet potato (OSP) with very high levels of vitamin A have been conventionally bred to combat vitamin-A deficiency in regions of Africa where sweet potato is a staple food. Studies have shown OSP improves vitamin-A status in young African children. Beginning in 2007, pilot programs successfully disseminated OSP to more than 24,000 households in Uganda and Mozambique. The project led to substantial substitution of OSP for nonbiofortified varieties in the cultivated areas devoted to OSP production. As a result, the intake of OSP, and thus vitamin A, increased for young children, older children, and women. Vitamin A intakes as much as doubled in some of these groups.

Sources: HarvestPlus 2010, Low et al. 2007, and Hotz et al. 2011.

However, by providing 30–50 percent of the daily nutrient requirement, biofortified crops can significantly improve public health in countries where hidden hunger is widespread (poor consumers in many cases will already be consuming about 50 percent of the estimated average requirements). Transgenic approaches can be used to improve the nutrient content of crops where natural variation in germplasm is limited. However, transgenic crops also face more regulatory hurdles compared to their conventionally bred counterparts. Whether conventionally or transgenically bred, biofortified crops should shift significant numbers of people that are receiving a little less than their estimated nutrient requirement, into a state of nutritional adequacy, for that nutrient.

Fourth, nutritionists now focus on the -9-to-24-month age group, when micronutrients are crucial for healthy development. Infants consume relatively low amounts of staple foods and yet have relatively higher micronutrient requirements, making biofortification's contribution to micronutrient adequacy in this group limited. There are exceptions; due to the particularly high vitamin-A content of many OSP varieties, regular consumption of these by the mother could contribute substantially to vitamin-A intakes of breastfed children 6–23 months of age. In Mozambique and Uganda, a HarvestPlus project also showed substantially improved vitamin A intakes from OSP in children aged 6–35 months (see Box 3).

However, researchers need to better understand biofortification's potential impact on the -9-to-24-month age group through the mother's micronutrient status *going into* pregnancy, when her micronutrient requirements substantially increase. This micronutrient status could be better for mothers who have consumed biofortified crops from adolescence, or even earlier.

Institutionalizing Biofortification as a Sustainable Strategy to Address Hidden Hunger

While substantial progress has been made to date in breeding and testing biofortified food crops, agricultural donors have been the primary investors in biofortification research. Increasing the efficiency of breeding biofortified crop varieties by doing more research on the key plant genes that (1) drive translocation of minerals from soils through the plant to seeds, and (2) are responsible for synthesis of vitamins in seeds will help in bring more agricultural decisionmakers on board. Moreover, research strategies that can leverage larger impacts should be supported. For example, most biofortification breeding efforts are directed at increasing the levels of selected minerals and vitamins. There is promising evidence, however, that breeding for prebiotics (nondigestible food ingredients that have health benefits) could greatly improve absorption and use of micronutrients (Bouis and Welch 2010).

This will pave the way for scaling up biofortification to reach millions, rather than just thousands, of households. Reaching these millions will require (a) integrating agriculture and nutritional platforms to fund and implement food-based approaches to reducing malnutrition, as was done in the Scaling-Up Nutrition framework and similar initiatives; (b) creating widespread demand for more nutritious crops and foods; and (c) building institutional capacity for developing and delivering nutrient-rich crops and foods with the right mix of partners to ensure the sustainability of this strategy.

Biofortification has distinct advantages that can complement other traditional approaches to improving nutrition. As more evidence emerges that nutritionally enhanced staple foods can cost-effectively alleviate crucial micronutrient deficiencies cost-effectively, biofortification will emerge as an agriculture-based strategy that could help considerably in meeting the nutritional needs of malnourished communities throughout the world.

References

Bouis, H. E., P. Eozenou, and A. Rahman. 2011. "Food Prices, Household Income, and Resource Allocation: Socioeconomic Perspectives on Their Effects on Dietary Quality and Nutritional Status," *Food and Nutrition Bulletin* 32 (1): s14–s23.

Bouis, H. E., C. Hotz, B. McClafferty, J. V. Meenakshi, and W. H. Pfeiffer. 2011. "Biofortification: A New Tool to Reduce Micronutrient Malnutrition." Supplement, *Food and Nutrition Bulletin* 32 (1): 31S-40S.

Bouis, H. E., and R. M. Welch. 2010. "Biofortification—a Sustainable Agricultural Strategy for Reducing Micronutrient Malnutrition in the Global South." *Crop Science* 50 (2): S1–S13.

Brown, K. H. 1991. "The Importance of Dietary Quality versus Quantity for Weanlings in Less Developed Countries: A Framework of Discussion." *Food and Nutrition Bulletin* 13: 86–92.

Cakmak, I. 2008. "Enrichment of Cereal Grains with Zinc: Agronomic or Genetic Biofortification?" *Plant Soil* 302:1–17.

DaMatta, F. M., A. Grandis, B. C. Arenque, and M. S. Buckeridge. 2010. "Impacts of Climate Changes on Crop Physiology and Food Quality," *Food Research International* 43 (7): 1814–1823.

HarvestPlus, *Disseminating Orange-Fleshed Sweet Potato: Findings from a HarvestPlus Project in Mozambique and Uganda*. Washington, DC: HarvestPlus, 2010.

Hoddinott, J., J. A. Maluccio, J. R. Behrman, R. Flores, and R. Martorell. 2008. "Effect of a Nutrition Intervention during Early Childhood on Economic Productivity in Guatemalan Adults." *Lancet* 371: 411–16.

Hotz, C., C. Loechl, A. de Brauw, P. Eozenou, D. Gilligan, M. Moursi, B. Munhaua, P. van Jaarsveld, A. Carriquiry, and J. V. Meenakshi. 2011. "A Large-Scale Intervention to Introduce Orange Sweet Potato in Rural Mozambique Increases Vitamin A Intakes among Children and Women." *British Journal of Nutrition*, 1–14.

Loladze, I. 2002. "Rising Atmospheric CO2 and Human Nutrition: Toward Globally Imbalanced Plant Stoichiometry?" *Trends in Ecology & Evolution* 17: 457–461.

Nelson, G. C., M. W. Rosegrant, A. Palazzo, I. Gray, C. Ingersoll, R. Robertson, S. Tokgoz, T. Zhu, T. B. Sulser, C. Ringler, S. Msangi, and L. You. 2010. *Food Security, Farming, and Climate Change to 2050*. Washington, DC: International Food Policy Research Institute.

Low, J. W., M. Arimond, N. Osman, B. Cunguara, F. Zano, and D. Tschirley. 2007. "A Food-Based Approach Introducing Orange-Fleshed Sweet Potatoes Increased Vitamin A Intake and Serum Retinol Concentrations in Young Children in Rural Mozambique." *Journal of Nutrition* 137 (5): 1320–1327.

Meenakshi, J.V. , N. L. Johnson, V. M. Manyong, H. DeGroote, J. Javelosa, D. R. Yanggen, F. Naher, C. Gonzalez, J. García, and E. Meng. 2010. "How Cost-Effective Is Biofortification in Combating Micronutrient Malnutrition? An Ex Ante Assessment." *World Development* 38 (1): 64–75.

Msangi, S., T. B. Sulser, A. Bouis, D. Hawes, and M. Batka. 2010. *Integrated Economic Modeling of Global and Regional Micronutrient Security*. HarvestPlus Working Paper 5. Washington, DC: HarvestPlus.

WHO (World Health Organization) and FAO (Food and Agriculture Organization of the United Nations). 2006. *Guidelines on Food Fortification with Micronutrients*. Geneva.

Chapter 11

Responding to Health Risks along the Value Chain

Pippa Chenevix Trench, Clare Narrod, Devesh Roy, and Marites Tiongco

In developing countries, consumption of unsafe food and water is one of the major causes of preventable illness and death. It exacerbates malnutrition; the spread of food- and water-borne diseases; and any associated economic losses to individuals, families, and society. Impaired health leads to reduced labor productivity and lower returns to schooling and training. It impacts livelihoods in both the short and long term. Safe food is not a luxury; it is an essential component of food security.

There are three factors that drive increasing health risks in food and water along the value chain:

1. shifts in consumption patterns, which are often linked to increasing incomes, toward perishable and processed foods that are highly susceptible to food-safety risks as they move along the value chain prior to consumption;

2. higher demand for cheap foods to address food insecurity for a growing global population, which leads to health risks related to intensification of production, increased dependency on chemical inputs, and increased risks of zoonoses and emerging zoonotic diseases and pandemics, such as swine flu; and

3. increases in urbanization, which lead to greater anonymity along the value chain—and therefore fewer incentives for individuals and institutions to invest in food safety—as well as elevated levels of contamination associated with wastewater irrigation.

The agrifood industry is subject to stringent safety requirements in the developed world, but most developing countries lack credible institutional mechanisms and affordable testing methods to monitor for hazards and ensure that highly perishable food products remain safe to consume as they move through the value chain.

This chapter is based on the authors' 2020 Conference Paper, *Responding to Health Risks along the Value Chain* (Washington, DC: International Food Policy Research Institute, 2011).

This chapter describes food safety risks along the value chain, identifies drivers of change, presents the risks posed to the poor by both food safety challenges
and recommends possible ways to address these risks. In particular, the chapter
underscores the use of risk-based analysis to craft effective food safety policies that
benefit both poor consumers and poor producers.[1]

Health Risks along the Value Chain

Health risks along agrifood value chains fall into three broad categories: microbiological hazards, physical and chemical contaminants, and occupational hazards.
While no less significant, the last category is not addressed in this chapter, which
focuses on a food-safety perspective.[2]

Microbiological hazards (includes food-borne pathogens and zoonoses)

The World Health Organization (WHO) estimates that in 2004 unsafe water,
lack of hygiene, and insufficient sanitation were responsible for 1.9 million deaths
and 64.2 million disability-adjusted life years (2009). Emerging zoonotic diseases
are likewise of major concern, particularly in developing countries. Such diseases
and their causes are often not recognized because of the lack of diagnostic capacity
along the value chain and poor infrastructure. The World Bank (2010) estimates
the costs of zoonotic diseases (including human and animal health service costs,
compensation for lost animals, and production and revenue losses to the livestock
sector) between 2000 and 2010 to be in excess of US$20 billion (or more than $200
billion with associated indirect costs).

Physical and chemical contaminants

Plant toxins are common in important food crops—such as cyanide in cassava or
tannin, vicine, and convicine in fava beans—and may cause specific diseases such
as favism, lathyrism, and konzo when consumed in large quantities over a prolonged
period of time. In smaller doses, these toxins can reduce micronutrient intake and
diminish immunity and growth in infants and children. Mycotoxins, including
aflatoxins and fuminosins, are toxic fungal byproducts thought to affect 25 percent
of the world's food crops. Aflatoxin has been listed as a Class A carcinogen that

---

1. This chapter uses terminology, such as health risks, risk analysis, and risk assessment, in a broad
literary sense intended for a lay reader rather than the tightly specified definitions as prescribed by
the Codex Alimentarius Commission.

2. From an occupational perspective, agriculture is one of the most hazardous sectors worldwide,
with agricultural workers exposed to extreme weather conditions, zoonoses, pesticide residues, and
agrochemical pollutants, among other risks.

causes liver cancer and has been associated with immune system suppression and stunting in children; however, it remains poorly monitored in developing countries (Gong et al. 2004).

Intensification of agriculture and expansion of markets for perishable foods have increased agribusinesses' reliance on pesticides, herbicides, and fungicides to maintain high agricultural productivity and reduce losses, both pre- and post-harvest. In urban and peri-urban areas, untreated wastewater used to irrigate food crops may be severely contaminated with chemicals. While export crops are generally carefully regulated for food safety, items for domestic consumption are less well scrutinized, and while exposure to agricultural chemicals is known to lead to varied health effects, including birth defects, blindness, cancer, and even death, their levels are weakly monitored in most developing countries. Additionally, poorly monitored food processing and preparation increasingly introduce additives and adulterants that present yet unquantified direct or indirect effects on human health.

Drivers of Change to Improve Food Safety

As income increases, consumer demand for safer and higher-quality food—in terms of willingness to pay more—also increases. Several studies in developed countries have found consumers willing to pay premiums for safer food. In contrast, research on demand for food safety in developing countries is scant, although there is some evidence that consumers will pay a premium if provided with credible information (Roy et al. 2010). Overall, demand for safer foods remains unproven among poorer consumers in developing countries, where coping with food insecurity is primarily focused on access to food rather than its quality or safety.

Private standards are also beginning to emerge, driven by supermarkets and modern value chains, in large part to compete with traditional retail markets and create a competitive advantage over other suppliers and retailers. These standards still only reach a limited number of consumers in most developing countries. However, as consumer awareness grows, so does pressure on governments to revise regulatory systems along the value chain and enforce compliance with food safety regulations and standards (Ng'etich 2010).

Additional drivers of positive change in food safety include advances in contamination detection methods through improved institutional capacity and reduced costs of diagnostics. Increasing concerns about food safety have boosted research to uncover quicker, more cost-effective methods of detecting and addressing food safety risks. Examples include standardized methods of DNA "fingerprinting" of disease-causing bacteria isolated from both humans and food to quickly identify the source of outbreaks and nanotechnology that can test for a variety of food safety hazards.

Finally, international standards and trade restrictions play an increasingly important role in food safety. Government activism on food safety, in response to pressure from consumer groups, is a double-edged sword: international sanitary and phytosanitary standards, while useful for enforcement in certain circumstances, have been used as a nontariff trade barrier to control imports from foreign sources, including developing countries.

Challenges for the Poor

Food and water safety affects the livelihoods of poor producers and poor consumers through two major channels: (1) health and (2) market access. Poorly considered or rigid policies to improve food safety can perversely increase the vulnerability of both consumers and farmers to exposure from unsafe food or zoonoses. Delivery of safe food will ultimately require a combination of pull from markets and push from public health and regulatory bodies. The problems that arise from food and water safety concerns affect different actors in the value chain in different ways.

Challenges faced by smallholders: Safe food costs more to produce, process, and deliver than food that is not monitored. These costs could affect the poor in the least-developed countries asymmetrically, particularly where there are high fixed costs and especially when the costs are not matched with a commensurate premium for safer food. Studies on aggregate measures of costs of compliance have found the direct costs of compliance in developing countries are substantial in relation to the value of their exports. Against the relatively high costs of compliance, small-scale producers face four distinct problems.

- *How to produce safe food:* Studies consistently find it is medium and large producers that can access resources to meet international food safety standards, such as cold storage facilities for meat and dairy produce and clean storage facilities for staples. The challenges for smallholders become more pronounced in the face of fast-changing regulatory regimes worldwide.

- *How to be recognized as producing safe food:* Small- and medium-scale producers have difficulties guaranteeing that the products they produce meet mandated standards due to a number of factors, including stringent requirements (and costs) of recognized standards, lack of capacity to accurately diagnose and certify safe foods, lack of alignment of incentives along the value chain in delivery of food safety, regulatory failures, and the cost of meeting certification requirements.

- *How to be competitive with larger producers:* Large retailers often prefer to work with large-scale producers or their own production operations, which are inherently easier to monitor and regulate. In Kenya, large exporters reduced the proportion of fruit and vegetables sourced from small-scale farmers from 45 percent in the mid-1980s to just 18 percent by the late 1990s (Jaffee 1990; Dolan, Humphrey, and Harris-Pascal 1999). Smallholders lack the scale and organization to perform many of the actions necessary to be incorporated in high-value agriculture. These include quality control, handling, storage, and marketing.

- *How to deal with asymmetry of information about consumer demands and safety standards:* Information on health standards required by markets is often not accessible to smallholders, a challenge exacerbated by a lack of coordination in the value chains. The exclusion of smallholders from high-value markets could also reflect a lack of awareness regarding market requirements, which could be magnified by smallholders' remoteness.

Challenges faced by consumers: When combined with inadequate implementation and regulation, increased food safety standards can actually have a negative effect on the health of the poor in a number of ways.

- Poor consumers cannot afford the premiums for food safety.

- Poor consumers could end up eating unsafe food if higher-safety or higher-quality products are sorted into the high-value export market, reserving low-quality contaminated food for the poorest consumers.

- Many health risks related to food safety along the value chain are chronic rather than acute, so they are less visible and have less priority, whereas food insecurity focuses on immediate access to enough food.

- Poor people are less likely to receive adequate or timely treatment for ailments caused by consumption of unsafe food and water.

- Poor people are less likely to have credible information pertinent for choosing safe food.

Significant challenges faced by other value-chain actors: Small-scale traders are largely neglected by studies on the impacts of health risks along the value chain. Little is known about their socioeconomic and livelihood status or the impact of food safety issues on them. Vertical integration and food-safety-related changes in procurement systems driven by large-scale markets and export markets will impact smaller actors throughout the value chain who do not have the advantages of economies of scale.

A Modified Risk Analysis Approach

Faced with uncertainty about outbreaks from unsafe food and adoption of control measures, decisionmakers are increasingly using analysis based on probability theory to help them undertake regulatory actions to prevent (or reduce) the incidence of disease.

In developing countries, the prevalence of many hazards is poorly understood, due in large part to the difficulty and cost of monitoring for hazards that are not evenly distributed in time and space. Without understanding the prevalence of a particular hazard along the value chain, it is difficult to identify the most cost-effective measures to reduce health risks. Quantifying the economic impacts of food-borne and animal diseases on human health and livelihoods is likewise important in order to assess the technological feasibility of the risk-reduction strategies.

Standard risk analysis techniques tailored to developed countries often do not take into account the diversity of actors in value chains in developing countries or the importance of socioeconomic factors that constrain behavior changes. A modified risk analysis framework (see Figure 1) integrates a traditional risk assessment for both food and plant and animal health and the evaluation of risk-management options with other behavioral factors that may affect the adoption of risk-reduction strategies, customizing the risk analysis for the developing-country context.

Once the costs and benefits of risk-reduction measures are measured, a cost-effectiveness analysis can be conducted to understand the tradeoffs of the risk-reduction methods available and help with risk-management decisions. Finally, impact evaluation of the effects that different strategies have on health and livelihoods in trials is assessed. Decisionmakers can weigh the available options for risk reduction in terms of efficiency, technological feasibility, and practicality at critical points along the value chain.[3]

Responding to Health Risks along the Value Chain

Adopt risk-based analyses. Significant gaps remain in our knowledge of the magnitude of health risks in developing countries and in terms of cost-effective approaches to mitigate such risks from farm to fork. Risk-based analyses allow for more nuanced

---

3. Results from the application of this model in the cases of aflatoxin contamination of groundnuts in Mali and maize in Kenya are available at http://programs.ifpri.org/afla/afla.asp.

Figu Re 1   Modified risk analysis framework

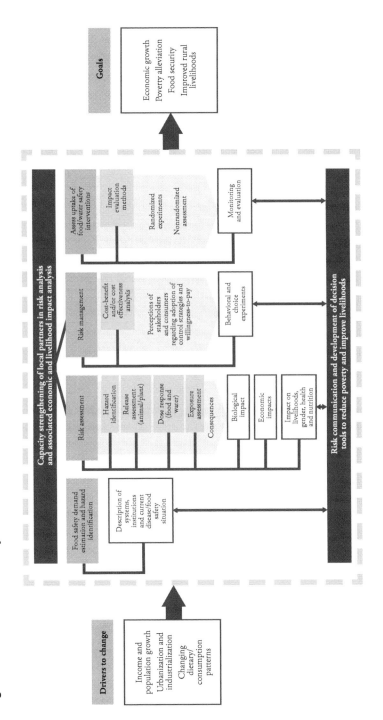

Source: Narrod et al. 2009.

approaches to health risks along the value chain. They are targeted and take into account the political, social, and economic feasibility of interventions as well as impacts on the health and livelihoods of the poor.

Respond to market failures. While private standards are driving better food standards for export markets, they cannot be relied on to ensure the delivery of safe food to poorer consumers in the least-developed countries. Governments have a key role to play in ensuring delivery of safe food, through regulation and oversight (through financial and legal sanctions), even where government resources are scarce. Governments can take the following actions to give consumers the protection that markets do not:

- Support and promote collective marketing groups among small-scale farmers. Collective action, such as rural producer organizations and cooperatives, can provide an important means to address cost constraints for small-scale producers. Contracts between producer groups and retail organizations that place a value on food safety standards can help reduce fixed costs of production and marketing (the dairy cooperatives in India provide a concrete example). Such collective action, however, requires significant inputs and up-front effort to support local capacity and to maintain the networks and relationships needed to ensure consistent food safety practices along the value chain. Contract farming also typically only applies to a small segment of the smallholder sector.

- Identify where there is potential for market failure and the need for a public-health-driven approach. Awareness campaigns and the dissemination of food safety education and knowledge are public goods that require public investment.

- Government regulation and oversight, as well as public information campaigns, are also essential to providing the drivers for technological innovation to reduce the costs of producing and delivering food that is safe to eat.

- Respond to government failures. Governments frequently lack the resources and capacity to deliver solutions that are cost-effective and appropriate to local conditions. Where effects of poor food safety are chronic and not readily visible, governments may lack political incentives to invest in immediate action. There are several ways to respond to these government failures:

  » Promote greater activism by civil society, consumer watchdog organizations, and other organizations that can hold government accountable. Such activism also creates greater incentives for producers to address food safety concerns, where food is sold through the markets.

» Information campaigns require a dynamic relationship between governments and civil society. Civil society and consumer organizations need to be informed and strengthened, with information made available in public places from schools to clinics to the market place.

» Finally, there must be greater integration of public health and agricultural departments within government.

Engage stakeholders in the value-chain approach. Solutions to food safety and health risks facing the poor in developing countries need to take into account the social, political, and economic realities of the market and stakeholders along the value chain. Important stakeholders include small-scale producers, traders, handlers, importers and exporters, retailers, consumers, international and multinational trade and health institutions, and the government institutions responsible for support and oversight of the agrifood industry and public health.

Concluding Remarks

Food safety policy in developing countries is, unfortunately, a double-edged sword: poor farmers are most vulnerable to losing market access when food safety requirements are tightened due to increased costs of compliance; poor consumers—particularly children and other high-risk groups—have the most to gain from access to safe, high-value agricultural products. Policymakers must look for solutions that incentivize low-cost, safe food production through technical and organizational investments, and inform both producers and consumers of the risks associated with poor food safety, which will ultimately drive demand for access to not just food but safe food.

References

Dolan, C. J. Humphrey, and C. Harris-Pascal. 1999. *Horticulture Commodity Chains: The Impact of UK Markets on African Fresh Vegetable Industry.* Institute of Development Studies Working Paper 96. Sussex, England, UK: University of Sussex.

Gong, Y., A. Hounsa, S. Egal, P. C. Turner, A. E. Sutcliffe, A. J. Hall, K. Cardwell, and C. P. Wild. 2004. "Postweaning Exposure to Aflatoxin Results in Impaired Child Growth: A Longitudinal Study in Benin, West Africa." *Environmental Health Perspectives* 112 (13): 1334–1338.

Jaffee, S. 1990. *Exporting High Value Food Commodities: Success Stories from Developing Countries.* World Bank Discussion Paper 198. Washington, DC: World Bank.

Narrod, C., M. Tiongco, D. Roy, M. Torero, D. Orden, E. Birol, A. Viceisza, D. Asare-Marfo, and Y. Yakhchilikov. 2009. *Food and Water Safety*. Washington, DC: International Food Policy Research Institute.

Ng'etich, J. 2010. "Alarm Over 2.3m Bags of Bad Maize in Market." *Daily Nation Newspaper*, November 26.

Roy, D., E. Birol, K. Deffner, and B. Karandikar. 2010. "Developing Country Consumers' Demand for Food Safety and Quality: Is Mumbai Ready for Certified and Organic Fruits?" In *Choice Experiments in Developing Countries: Implementation, Challenges and Policy Implications*, edited by J. W. Bennett and E. Birol. Cheltenham, England, UK: Edward-Elgar Publishing.

WHO (World Health Organization). 2009. *Global Health Risks: Mortality and Burden of Disease Attributable to Selected Major Risks*. Geneva.

World Bank. 2010. World dataBank: World Development Indicators and Global Development Finance. Accessed January 19. http://databank.worldbank.org/ddp/home.do.

Chapter 12

Agriculture-Associated Diseases: Adapting Agriculture to Improve Human Health

John McDermott and Delia Grace

Agriculture is critical for human welfare, providing food, employment, income, and assets. In the past, agricultural research and development largely focused on improving production, productivity, and profitability of agricultural enterprises. Nutrition and other benefits of agriculture were not always optimized, while the negative impacts on health, well-being, and the environment were often ignored. This was especially problematic for livestock systems, with especially complex negative and positive impacts on human health and well-being.

An important negative effect of agricultural intensification is disease. Highly pathogenic avian influenza (HPAI) is a notorious example of a disease that was fostered by intensified agricultural production and spread through lengthened poultry value chains and the global movement of people and animals. Large-scale irrigation projects, designed to increase agriculture productivity, have created ecosystems conducive to schistosomiasis and Rift Valley fever.

The responses to disease threats are often compartmentalized. Instead of analyzing the tradeoffs between agricultural benefits and risks, the agriculture sector focuses on productivity, while the health sector focuses on managing disease. A careful look at the epidemiology of diseases associated with agriculture, and past experience of control efforts, shows that successful management must be systems-based rather than sectorally designed.

What Are Agriculture-Associated Diseases?

Any disease related to agrifood value chains can be considered agriculture-associated. Such diseases may be associated with agriculture inputs, primary agricultural

This chapter is based on the authors' 2020 Conference Brief, *Agriculture-Associated Diseases: Adapting Agriculture to Improve Human Health* (Washington, DC: International Food Policy Research Institute, 2011).

production, post-harvest processing and handling along marketing chains, or even final preparation by the consumer. The category also includes diseases influenced by ecosystem changes driven by food production (for example, large dams) and changes associated with agroecoystem incursion into natural ecosystems (for example, harvesting wildlife). Hence, a broad definition includes human diseases present or emerging in agroecosystems, which are linked directly or indirectly to practices in agrifood chains or agriculture. This includes diseases associated not only with livestock but also with other domestic and peri-domestic animals (such as rabies and leishmaniasis) and not only zoonotic diseases of livestock but also non-zoonotic diseases that have emerged from animals (such as HIV/AIDS and SARS).

The link between agriculture and disease has long been established. This chapter examines the range of agriculture-associated diseases to discover commonalities that can be leveraged to achieve better health outcomes. To frame the discussion, Box 1 presents a typology of four categories of these diseases based on causation and transmission pathways, ranking them by overall impact on human health as measured in disability-adjusted life years (DALYs); DALYs are used to measure the healthy years of life lost due to premature death and disability produced. As with any typology of disease, there are overlaps and ambiguities; the categories are not intended to be absolute but rather to have pragmatic relevance for policy and practice.

Why Do Agriculture-Associated Diseases Matter—and to Whom?

As well as sickening and killing billions of people each year, these diseases damage economies, societies, and environments. While there is no metric that captures the full cost of disease, assessments of specific disease outbreaks suggest the scale of potential impacts. For example, the SARS epidemic cost US$50–100 billion; the potential costs of an avian influenza pandemic are estimated at US$3 trillion (World Bank 2010). These findings have stimulated rich and middle-income countries to invest heavily in a global program of pandemic prevention and risk reduction.

In low-income countries, the total disease burden is much higher than in high-income countries, and the share of infectious and respiratory diseases is more than ten times greater. Zoonoses and diseases recently emerged from animals constitute 20 percent of the infectious and respiratory disease burden (which in turn accounts for 40 percent or the total burden) whereas in high-income countries zoonoses and diseases recently emerged from animals constitute 3 percent of the infectious and respiratory disease burden, which is only 3 percent of the total burden. The direct economic, social, and environmental costs of these diseases are probably proportionate to the adverse health impacts: for example, fungal toxins (mycotoxins) in

Box 1   Agriculture-Associated Diseases

Zoonoses and emerging infectious disease. At least 61 percent of all human pathogens are zoonotic (transmissible between animals and man), and zoonoses make up 75 percent of emerging infectious diseases. A new disease emerges every four months; many are trivial, but HIV, SARS, and avian influenza illustrate the huge potential impacts. *Zoonoses and zoonotic diseases recently emerged from animals are responsible for 8 percent of the total disease burden in low-income countries.*

Food-associated disease. Diarrhea is one of the top three infectious diseases in most poor countries, killing an estimated 1.4 million children each year. Between 33 and 90 percent of diarrhea is attributed to food, and animal source food is the most risky. More than 90 percent of food sickness is caused by biological pathogens. Toxins and chemical hazards associated with food are also important health threats, and in many cases can be prevented only by farm-level intervention. *Foodborne disease is responsible for at least 4 percent of the disease burden in low-income countries.*

Water-associated disease. These include diseases spread by contaminated irrigation water—such as cholera, cryptosporidiosis, and chemical intoxication—and those that breed within irrigation and water storage systems, such as schistosomiasis and malaria. Malaria alone kills 1.1 million people annually. For most diseases, water is only one contributing factor. *Around 6 percent of the disease burden in least-developed countries is attributed to water-associated disease.*

Occupational disease and drug resistance. People working in agrifood systems are directly exposed to a range of biological, chemical, and physical hazards. The use of antibiotics in farm animals is known to contribute to the crisis of drug resistant bacteria in human medicine, although there is debate about its importance and the best way of tackling it. *The contribution to disease burden of this category has not been comprehensively assessed; it appears to be an order of magnitude less than the other disease categories.*

Source: Grace and Jones 2011.

food lead to trade losses of up to US$1.2 billion a year. Indirect costs of disease are also important. Impaired human health lowers both labor productivity and human capital accumulation (as through schooling and training), worsening livelihood outcomes in both the short run and the long run. Malnutrition itself is responsible for 3 percent of the disease burden in low-income countries (WHO 2010). Malnutrition enhances vulnerability to disease and is, in turn, exacerbated by disease symptoms—leading, for example, to a 30-fold increase in the risk for death from diarrhea (Flint et al. 2005).

Diseases are influenced by socioeconomics, environments, and policies. There are two broad scenarios that characterize poor countries. At one extreme are neglected areas that lack even the most basic services; in these "cold spots" diseases that are controlled elsewhere persist with strong links to poverty, malnutrition, and powerlessness. At the other extreme are areas of rapid intensification, where new and often unexpected disease threats emerge in response to rapidly changing practices and interactions between people, animals, and ecosystems. These areas are hot spots for the emergence of new diseases (of which 75 percent are zoonotic). They are also more vulnerable to food-borne disease, as agricultural supply chains diversify and outpace workable regulatory mechanisms.

Metrics, Partnerships, and Systems Approaches to Solving Complex Problems

Improved Metrics

What cannot be measured cannot be effectively and efficiently managed. Addressing agriculture-associated disease requires assessing and prioritizing its impacts, by measuring not only the multiple burdens of disease but also the multiple costs and benefits of potential interventions—across health, agriculture, and other sectors. For assessing the human health burden, the DALY is the standard metric. There are established methodologies, such as cost analysis and computable general equilibrium models, to measure the cost of illness to households and to the public health sector, as well as the economic costs of livestock disease to agriculture, food industry, and other sectors such as tourism. Costs in terms of non-marketed goods and services (such as loss of ecosystem services) can be estimated through willingness to pay and other indirect methods. (Sporadic and potential diseases are better assessed through decision analysis.)

But these assessment tools and results have rarely been integrated to yield a comprehensive assessment of the health, economic, and environmental costs of a particular disease. When they are brought together, surprising insights can emerge regarding the true impacts of disease and who bears them, with implications for

---

Box 2   Brucellosis control in Mongolia

In Mongolia, a cost-benefit analysis of brucellosis control, examining both medical and veterinary impacts, found that the public health sector reaps only about 10 percent of the benefits (Roth et al. 2003). Brucellosis control would thus appear less attractive than other disease control expenditure options, in an analysis based solely on DALYs averted. But when the benefits for the livestock sector were included, and the costs shared proportionally between the public health and the agricultural sector, the control of brucellosis actually offered a net gain for both sectors.

---

appropriate policy responses. An example comes from Mongolia, where brucellosis control was shown to be cost-effective from an integrated perspective (see Box 2).

Improved metrics for estimating the full costs of disease would open new approaches for the control of agriculture-associated diseases in developing countries. But even with better assessment tools, there remains the challenge of using the results to inform policy decisions. Decisionmakers require more than metrics: they need clear evidence on control options and the expected health and economic returns, and they need to consider the sociopolitical factors that affect the feasibility, sustainability, and acceptability of implementation. In the case of brucellosis, these assessments were relatively straightforward. For other agriculture-associated diseases, however, there are high levels of uncertainty regarding epidemiology, impacts, and control options. (This is true especially for emerging diseases and diseases sensitive to new drivers, such as climate change and evolving agroecosystems and food chains.) Other diseases have persisted despite medical interventions—especially the neglected tropical zoonoses—indicating a need to tackle the underlying determinants of disease, such as poverty, inequity, lack of information, and powerlessness.

Stronger Partnerships
Compiling convincing evidence is only the first step in shaping policy. Strong partnerships and high trust will be needed among researchers, stakeholders, and policymakers. Policy discussions must go beyond specific control measures to examine the incentives that underpin behavior and behavior change.

Systems Approaches
The complexities of agriculture-associated diseases call for more integrated and comprehensive approaches to analyze and address them, as envisioned in One

---

Box 3 0 ne health and ecohealth

One Health focuses on the integration of human medicine, veterinary medicine, and environmental science. The One Health approach has been defined as the collaborative effort of multiple disciplines to attain optimal health for people, animals, and our environment.

EcoHealth, with origins in ecosystem health, has been defined as systemic, participatory approaches to understanding and promoting health and well-being in the context of social and ecological interactions (Waltner-Toews 2009).

The two approaches have much in common and are increasingly aligned; both emphasize multidisciplinary action and the importance of agriculture and ecosystem-based interventions.

Health and EcoHealth perspectives (see Box 3). These integrated approaches offer a broad framework for understanding and addressing complex disease: they bring together key elements of human, animal, and ecosystem health; and they explicitly address the social, economic, and political determinants of health. Both of these global approaches recognize agriculture- and ecosystem-based interventions as a key component of multidisciplinary approaches for managing diseases. For example, food-borne disease requires management throughout the field-to-fork risk pathway. Zoonoses in particular cannot be controlled, in most cases, while disease remains in the animal reservoir. Similarly, agriculture practices that create health risks require farm-level intervention.

Systemic One Health and EcoHealth approaches require development and testing of methods, tools, and approaches to better support management of the diseases associated with agriculture. The potential impacts justify the substantial investment required. An ex ante assessment in Ghana evaluated an integrated package of risk-based measures relating to the use of wastewater for irrigation; it was judged capable of averting up to 90 percent of an estimated 12,000 DALYs, at an overall cost of less than US$100 per averted DALY (IFPRI and ILRI 2010).

Policy Implications

Better Information

As a basis for framing sound policies, information is needed on the multiple (that is, cross-sectoral) burdens of disease and the multiple costs and benefits of control, as well as the sustainability, feasibility, and acceptability of control options. An example of cross-disciplinary research that effectively influenced policy is the case of smallholder dairy in Kenya. In light of research by ILRI and partners, assessing both public health risks and poverty impacts of regulation, there was a dramatic shift in policy and regulation. This shift stopped pending legislation outlawing the selling of milk through the informal milk sector and officially recognized and supported the informal sector by establishing a system of training and certification for small-scale market agents. Not only did this improve the quality and safety of milk but it also led to economic benefits later estimated at US$26 million per year. This positive change required new collaboration among research groups, the government, nongovernmental organizations, and the private sector, as well as new ways of working. This policy shift is appropriate for the current context of milk marketing in Kenya and will be reviewed as this marketing chain evolves.

Many agriculture-associated diseases are characterized by complexity, uncertainty, and high potential impact. They call for both *analytic* thinking, to break problems into manageable components that can be tackled over time, and *holistic* thinking, to recognize patterns and wider implications as well as potential benefits.

The analytic approach is illustrated in the new decision-support tool developed to address Rift Valley fever in Kenya. In savannah areas of east Africa, climate events trigger a cascade of changes in environment and vectors, causing outbreaks of Rift Valley fever among livestock and, ultimately, humans. Improving information on step-wise events can lead to better decisions about whether, when, where, and how to institute control (Consultative Group for RVF Decision Support 2010).

An example of holistic thinking is pattern recognition applied to disease dynamics, recognizing that emerging diseases have multiple drivers. A synoptic view of apparently unrelated health threats—the unexpected establishment of chikungunya fever in northern Italy, the sudden appearance of West Nile virus in North America, the increasing frequency of Rift Valley fever epidemics in the Arabian Peninsula, and the emergence of Bluetongue virus in northern Europe—strengthens the suspicion that a warming climate is driving disease expansion generally.

Complex problems often benefit from a synergy of various areas of expertise and approaches. The Foresight groups successfully bring together experts in health, environment, agriculture, and social development to look at emerging issues. (See, for example, the Foresight group in the United Kingdom at www.bis.gov.uk/foresight.) Complex problems also require a longer-term view, informed by the understanding that short-term solutions can have unintended effects that lead to long-term problems—as in the case of agricultural intensification fostering health threats. Not every problem requires this broad-spectrum approach, so a first task is to identify specific problems that call for integrative solutions.

New Institutions

New, integrative ways of working on complex problems, such as One Health and EcoHealth, require new institutional arrangements. The agriculture, environment, and health sectors are not designed to promote integrated, multidisciplinary approaches to complex, cross-sectoral problems. Many exciting initiatives provide examples of successful institutional collaboration. For short-term outbreaks, joint task forces may be adequate, as in preventing an avian influenza outbreak. For longer-term planning and assessment, stronger cross-sectoral mechanisms may be required: joint animal and human health units; integrated knowledge management and information sharing; and integrated training programs. Institutional arrangements must carefully consider incentives for changing behavior, tailored to local contexts, needs, and cultures. Given the global impact of zoonoses and emerging diseases, international institutional arrangements are also critical. Such arrangements for better information sharing and coordinated action through WHO, FAO, and OIE have begun in response to the SARS and avian influenza epidemics. More attention needs to be paid to how low-income countries can effectively and appropriately participate in these coordinated global arrangements.

Conclusion

Agriculture and health are intimately linked. Many diseases have agricultural roots—food-borne diseases, water-associated diseases, many zoonoses, most emerging infectious diseases, and occupational diseases associated with agrifood chains. These diseases create an especially heavy burden for poor countries, with far-reaching impacts. This chapter views agriculture-associated disease as the dimension of public health shaped by the interaction among humans, animals, and agroecosystems. This conceptual approach presents new opportunities for shaping agriculture to improve health outcomes, in the short and long term.

Understanding the multiple burdens of disease is a first step in its rational management. As agriculture-associated diseases occur at the interface of human health, animal health, agriculture, and ecosystems, addressing them often requires systems-based thinking and multidisciplinary approaches. These approaches, in turn, require new ways of working and institutional arrangements. Several promising initiatives demonstrate convincing benefits of new ways of working across disciplines, despite the considerable barriers to cooperation.

References

Consultative Group for RVF Decision Support. 2010. "Decision-Support Tool for Prevention and Control of Rift Valley Fever Epizootics in the Greater Horn of Africa." *American Journal of Tropical Medicine and Hygiene* 83 (2 Supplement): 75–85.

Grace, D., and Jones. 2011. *Zoonoses: Wildlife Domestic Animal Interactions.* A report to DFID. Nairobi and London: International Livestock Research Institute and Royal Veterinary College.

Flint, J., et al. 2005. "Estimating the Burden of Acute Gastroenteritis, Foodborne Disease, and Pathogens Commonly Transmitted by Food: An International Review." *Clinical Infectious Diseases* 41: 698–704.

IFPRI (International Food Policy Research Institute) and ILRI (International Livestock Research Institute). 2010. *Agriculture for Improved Nutrition and Health.* Washington, DC, and Nairobi, Kenya.

Roth, F., et al. 2003. "Human Health Benefits from Livestock Vaccination for Brucellosis: Case Study." *World Health Organization Bulletin* 8 (12): 867–876.

Waltner-Toews, D. 2009., "Eco-Health: A Primer for Veterinarians." *Canadian Veterinary Journal* 50 (5): 519–521.

VSF (Vétérinaires sans Frontières/Veterinarians without Borders). 2010. *One Health for One World: A Compendium of Case Studies.* Victoria, British Columbia, Canada.

WHO (World Health Organization). 2010. *Global Burden of Disease.* Geneva.

World Bank. 2010. *People, Pathogens and our Planet: One Health Approach for Controlling Zoonotic Disease.* Washington, DC.

Chapter 13

Do Health Investments Improve Agricultural Productivity? Lessons from Agricultural Household and Health Research

Paul E. McNamara, John M. Ulimwengu, and Kenneth L. Leonard

T he link between good health and economic prosperity is well established and can be detected in numerous measures, such as increased income, wages, efficiency, and productivity. While the link can readily be seen in descriptive statistics, it is another matter to disentangle the precise nature of the connection. It is likely that causality runs in both directions, and both health and prosperity clearly are affected by numerous other variables.

A similar observation can be made for the link between health and increases in agricultural productivity. This chapter seeks to address a fundamental question: Does better health lead to higher rates of agricultural growth? Likely, yes, as a healthier farmer and farm household can devote more resources to farming. It is also likely that the household's greater productivity leads to higher levels of health because, among other things, the healthy farm family may achieve greater income and therefore be able to purchase more and better healthcare, which would lead to even higher productivity and so on, in a virtuous circle that also includes many other inputs and effects.

Despite the number of studies focusing on the links between health status and economic outcomes, very few focus on the contribution of improvements in health to agricultural growth. Given the need for long-term research and the paucity of high-quality data on the agricultural sector for most countries, this is largely unavoidable. This chapter reviews the literature related to health, healthcare, and agricultural productivity in an effort to identify such gaps. At both micro- and macro-levels, the literature does not provide a clear-cut answer to the chapter's

This chapter is based on the authors' IFPRI Discussion Paper (1012), *Do Health Investments Improve Agricultural Productivity? Lessons from Agricultural Household and Health Research.* (Washington, DC: International Food Policy Research Institute, 2011).

fundamental question: Do health investments improve agricultural productivity? Filling in the knowledge gaps could lead to more effective policy and interventions.

Linking Health, Healthcare, and Agricultural Outcomes

Statistics on various health input measures in Sub-Saharan Africa demonstrate a positive relationship between these measures and levels of agricultural value-added. The prevalence of child stunting, prevalence of underweight children, percentage of overall households with improved sanitation, and percentage of rural households with improved sanitation demonstrate a distinct connection between higher levels of agricultural value-added and better health status or health-system measures. This type of simple descriptive statistical relationship motivates much of the interest in exploring the link between health inputs and agricultural productivity. It is of policy relevance to know, for example, if a higher physician-to-person ratio in an area leads to better healthcare, if that care leads to better health, and if that improvement in health directly increases farmers' productivity.

That income and health are interrelated is beyond question. Higher-income countries have better health, and, as incomes grow across populations, their overall health improves. It is also widely known that agricultural productivity has histori-cally played an essential role in economic development. Increases in productivity in the agriculture sector release resources (primarily labor and low-cost food) for use in the nascent industrial sector. Some researchers have argued that education has a greater causal impact on agricultural productivity than does health (Huffman and Orazem 2007). Nonetheless, this process of economic development has always been accompanied by improved health.

There are important questions to be addressed by policymakers, practitioners, funders, and other stakeholders. What are the direction and amplitude of the rela-tionships among healthcare, health status, and productivity? What other variables are at play in the relationship between productivity and health? Empirical findings on the relationship between health conditions and wages, profit, or income are at best difficult to generalize (see Table 1 for a summary of coefficients reported in the literature). The review of empirical findings on the link between health and agriculture at the microlevel reveals a rather heterogeneous body of literature. Many researchers use health indicators that actually combine health and nutrition factors (such as caloric intake and BMI), and as a result the studies do not strictly provide evidence on the relationship between health and performance indicators. Many of the studies do not take account of the two-way causality between health and per-formance indicators, likely yielding biased estimates and inaccurate test statistics. Simple answers do not present themselves; stakeholders who ignore the complexity

TAb Le 1 **Summary of studies with estimated coefficients linking health to agricultural productivity**

Study author(s)	health variables	Estimated coefficients	agricultural productivity variables
Deolalikar (1988)	Calorie intake[ns]	Calorie intake[ns]	Market Wages
	Weight-for-height	Weight-for-height	Farm Output
		-0.06 (FE)	Market Wages
		0.07 (FE)[ns]	Farm Output
		0.66 (FE)	
		1.32 (FE)	
Kim et al. (1997)	Onchocercal Skin disease (OSD): binary variable (0 and 1)	i) Severe OSD	Daily Wages
		-0.159 (All)	
		-0.136 (Age 15-35)	
		ii) No OSD	
		0.185 (All)	
		-0.936 (Age 15-35)	
Behrman et al. (1997)	Calorie intake	i) <1.5 acres	Income
		0.34	
		ii) >=1.5 acres	
		0.22	
Croppenstedt and Muller (2000)	Body Mass Index (BMI)	2.7 (All)[ns]	Wages
		3.0 (Males)	
		2.2 (All)[ns]	
		3.6 (Males)	
		3.0 (Males)	
Strauss (1986)	Calorie intake	0.33	Output
Ayalew (2003)	Calorie intake	1.47 (IV)	Wages
		0.55 (FE)	
		0.21 (RE)[ns]	
Audibert and Etard (2003)	Schistosomiasis treatment: binary (0 and 1)	difference between the two groups because of treatment: 0.07 Kg/ha (Paddy) 0.26 Kg/ha/person-day	Yield
Fox et al. (2004)	HIV/AIDS infection: binary (0 and 1)	7.1 kg less tea leaf per plucking day	Productivity

Notes: ns = not significant; FE = fixed effects; RE = random effects; IV = instrumental variables estimator.

of these interrelationships put the effectiveness of their programs and projects—not to mention the improvement of farmers' well-being—at risk.

Distinguishing between Health and Healthcare

The most obvious problem in addressing the impact of healthcare on agricultural development is the divide between health and healthcare. There are many potential indicators of health, and they may have different effects on productivity. Since healthcare spending is only one of the factors that drive healthcare outcomes, such as mortality, it is impetuous to assume that healthcare spending will always increase agricultural productivity.

The evidence at the country and global level is mixed at best and, in some cases, suggests that healthcare interventions have no impact on income, much less on agricultural productivity. But these results may reflect limitations in research methods and the difficulties in dealing with an enormous array of variables. The evidence from some micro-level studies suggests that inexpensive health interventions can have a very large impact on labor productivity.

In the poorest countries, there is little debate about the role of public expenditure in health. In some poor countries, for example, incomes are so low that the cost to families of malaria prevention exceeds the benefit. Evidence suggests the existence of two groups of countries: those experiencing high incomes and high prevention and those experiencing low incomes and low prevention. The latter group is generally considered good ground for outside intervention.

Disentangling an Array of Health-Related Variables

The importance of health in promoting economic development has been forcefully stated by the World Health Organization's Commission on Macroeconomics and Health (Sachs 2001). However, economists and development policy analysts debate the commission's contentions and evidence, and the overall evidence of the impact of poor health on economic development appears to be mixed. Studies that attempt to explain intercountry differences in economic growth and productivity rates, for instance, have suggested that education, trade openness, savings, inflation, and the initial level of income, rather than health, are the key explanatory variables.

Studies from India and China suggest that healthcare expenditures had no impact on rural gross domestic product (GDP), agricultural GDP, or rural poverty (Fan, Hazell, and Thorat 2000; Zhang and Fan 2004). On the other hand, expenditures on roads, education, and agricultural research and development had strong positive impacts. Thus, while healthcare spending is necessary, it is not sufficient to improve health. Spending, such as investments in facilities, medicines, and doctors, may have little direct payoff if it is not associated with improvements in education or transportation. (Direct spending on health, such as vaccinations or iron supplements, might work independent of infrastructure.) However, investments in transportation or education by themselves would not lead to improvements in health either. Such investments—usually motivated by reasons other than health—will improve health when they are complemented by investments in facilities and doctors. The fact that these investments are tied to each other makes it difficult to measure the direct impact of health investments.

There is every reason to believe that spending on roads directly increases the value of existing public health facilities. In parts of rural Tanzania, improvements in roads have had a larger impact on healthcare access than improvements in health facilities because travel costs were one of the major impediments to access (Klemick, Leonard, and Masatu 2009). Based on several indicators, villages in Indonesia, the Philippines, and Sri Lanka participating in rural roads projects reported better access to health services compared with nonproject villages (Hettige 2006). Travel time to health services was three times lower in areas with project sites, and, since household members were more likely to travel to medical facilities by bicycle, car, or bus than by foot, improved roads were of great importance. Households in nonproject villages were twice as likely to use traditional healers or stay home during a medical emergency. Similar relationships between rural infrastructure and healthcare access have been found in Morocco, Vietnam, and elsewhere.

Choosing effective Investments

The positive relationship between health and agricultural productivity does not occur in isolation. Interventions and policies must take into account a wide array of variables. That being said, a single, wide-ranging, all-purpose initiative is not feasible due to the complexity and shifting nature of interrelationships. A breadth of interventions and policies is needed, and greater success will likely be achieved when each is undertaken with its potential relationship to the others in mind.

Focused, inexpensive micro-level health interventions are known to have an impact. The evidence from some micro-level studies suggests that inexpensive health interventions can have a very large impact on labor productivity. One study followed Indonesian rubber workers who were given 100 milligrams of iron per day for 60 days. Not only did their work effort improve during the intervention, but the increased earnings and nutritional intake enabled them to permanently increase their caloric intake, blood iron levels, and income. This is a remarkable transformation for an intervention with almost no cost (Basta et al. 1979).

Coordinated h ealthcare e ducation pr ograms a nd i nfrastructure pr ojects h old promise. It may seem self-evident that the coordination of various public and private initiatives yields more effective results in numerous areas, but projects often remain "siloed" in their respective sectors. The challenge here is administrative and bureaucratic. Capacity building in collaborative planning and implementation may hold promise.

Improved health during childhood can have a lasting impact on the level and rate of depreciation of human capital. Healthy children have better cognitive abilities and grow into taller and generally healthier adults. In particular, there is strong evidence that economic growth in early industrialized countries was associated with significantly increased caloric intake, which produced greater height and body mass index (Fogel 2004a, 2004b). In addition, healthy children learn more in school and are more likely to stay in school. Similarly, a study of Guatemalan boys who participated in a randomized nutrition intervention from conception through their first two years of life showed that they earned wages as adults that were 50 percent higher than those of nonparticipants (Hoddinott et al. 2008).

Concluding Remarks

The literature at both macro- and micro-levels presents some significant gaps. More research is needed to understand consumer perceptions and determinants of health production. Benchmarking the productivity effects of health by various health instruments, such as prevention (for example, immunization and screening); health protection (for example, water sanitation and precautions against specific diseases); and positive health education (for example, training farmers in the use of pesticides) represents a policy-relevant research agenda. What specific crops or groups of crops yield the highest productivity impact from health investments? Research-based responses to this and similar questions should help improve policy interventions.

If the poorest countries follow the development path of most industrialized economies, it is likely that increases in agricultural productivity will precede those of nonagricultural sectors. It would therefore be relevant to study the impact of health on agricultural productivity by looking for evidence that certain investments in health lead directly to increases in productivity. Such studies should provide microlevel evidence that specific investments in health can improve agricultural performance at the household level and therefore help spark agricultural productivity growth.

References

Audibert, M., and J.-F. Etard. 2003. "Productive Benefits after Investment in Health in Mali." *Economic Development and Cultural Change* 51: 760–782.

Ayalew, T. 2003. *The Nutrition–Productivity Link and the Persistence of Poverty.* Discussion Paper 2003–02. Antwerp, Belgium: Institute of Development Policy and Management, University of Antwerp.

Basta, S. S., M. S. Soekirman, D. Karyadi, and N. S. Scrimshaw. 1979. "Iron Deficiency Anemia and the Productivity of Adult Males in Indonesia." *American Journal of Clinical Nutrition* (32): 916–925.

Behrman, J. R., A. D. Foster, and M. R. Rosenzweig. 1997. "The Dynamics of Agricultural Production and the Calorie-Income Relationship." *Journal of Econometrics* 77: 187–208.

Croppenstedt, A., and C. Muller. 2000. "The Impact of Farmers' Health and Nutrition Status on Their Productivity and Efficiency: Evidence from Ethiopia." *Economic Development and Cultural Change* 48: 475–502.

Deolalikar, A. B. 1988. "Nutrition and Labor Productivity In Agriculture: Estimates For Rural South India." *Review of Economics and Statistics* 70: 406–413.

Fan, S., P. Hazell, and S. Thorat. 2000. "Government Spending, Growth and Poverty in Rural India." *American Journal of Agricultural Economics* 82 (4): 1038–1051.

Fogel, R. W. 2004a. "Economic Growth, Population Theory, and Physiology: The Bearing of Long-Term Processes on the Making of Economic Policy." *American Economic Review* 84 (3): 369–95.

———. 2004b. "Health, Nutrition, and Economic Growth." *Economic Development and Cultural Change* 52 (3): 643–658.

Fox, M. P., S. Rosen, W. B. MacLeod, M. Wasunna, M. Bii, G. Foglia, and J. L. Simon. 2004. "The Impact of HIV/AIDS on Labour Productivity in Kenya." *Tropical Medicine and International Health* 9:318–324.

Hettige, H. 2006. *When Do Rural Roads Benefit the Poor and How?* Manila, the Philippines: Asian Development Bank.

Hoddinott, J., J. A. Maluccio, J. R. Behrman, R. Flores, and R. Martorell. 2008. "Effect of a Nutrition Intervention during Early Childhood on Economic Productivity in Guatemalan Adults." *The Lancet* 371 (610): 411–416.

Huffman, W. E., and P. F. Orazem. 2007. "Agriculture and Human Capital in Economic Growth: Farmers, Schooling and Nutrition." In *Handbook of Agricultural Economics*, edited by R. Evenson and P. Pingali. Vol. 3. Amsterdam: Elsevier.

Kim, A., A. Tandon, and A. Hailu. 1997. *Health and Labour Productivity: Economic Impact of Onchocercal Skin Disease.* Policy Research Working Paper 1836. Washington, DC: World Bank.

Klemick, H., K. L. Leonard, and M. C. Masatu. 2009. "Defining Access to Health Care: Evidence on the Importance of Quality and Distance in Rural Tanzania." *American Journal of Agricultural Economics* 91 (2): 347–358.

Sachs, J. D. 2001. *Macroeconomics and Health: Investing in Health for Economic Development.* Report of the Commission on Macroeconomics and Health. Geneva: World Health Organization.

Strauss, J. 1986. "Does Better Nutrition Raise Farm Productivity?" *Journal of Political Economy* 94: 297–320.

Zhang, X., and S. Fan. 2004. "How Productive Is Infrastructure? A New Approach and Evidence from Rural India." *American Journal of Agricultural Economics* 86 (2): 494–501.

Chapter 14

Two-Way Links between Health and Farm Labor

Kwadwo Asenso-Okyere, Catherine Chiang, Paul Thangata, and Kwaw S. Andam

Health issues are increasingly affecting household decisionmaking, farm labor, and agricultural productivity in developing countries. Similarly, certain agricultural development projects and practices that aid productivity (for example, the use of pesticides and the water harvesting techniques, storage structures, and dams involved with irrigation) can actually exacerbate the incidence of diseases in workers by increasing interactions with disease vectors and parasites. Failure to consider either the negative or positive health effects of certain farm practices or interventions can distort their impact; for example, an estimate of the real economic benefits of adopting pest-resistant crops or organic farming must take into account the positive health impacts accruing from decreased pesticide use.

Development practitioners must understand the relationship between health, farm labor, and agricultural productivity in order to design effective policies to maximize both farmers' well-being and agricultural production while minimizing any harmful interactions between them. To achieve this, the two-way linkages need to be assessed, and the specific impact pathways of a disease—including its effects on household decisionmaking, labor, and livelihoods—should be monitored.

Impacts of Disease on Farm Labor Productivity

When disease afflicts farmers, their productivity is reduced and they remain in poverty with an unacceptable standard of living. Three-quarters of the world's poor people live in rural areas, particularly in Asia and Africa, and depend on agriculture as their primary source of livelihood (Ravallion, Chen, and Sangraula 2007). The impact of severe or chronic illness on these households can be devastating.

The health of rural households is not only an issue of social welfare, however, but also a key factor in economic development. A productive agricultural sector

This chapter is based on the authors' IFPRI Food Policy Report, *Interactions between Health and Farm–Labor Productivity* (Washington, DC: International Food Policy Research Institute, 2011).

depends on a healthy agricultural workforce. As shown in Figure 1, farm productivity (measured in terms of agricultural value added per farm worker) is quite low in developing countries, which rely heavily on manual labor and have a high incidence of disease, compared with the productivity of high- and middle-income countries, which rely on farm machinery more than labor and have a substantially lower incidence of disease.

Short-Term Impacts: Loss of Labor, Time, and Assets

The more immediate and obvious effects of disease on agricultural households can be catastrophic. They are best understood along three parameters: (1) loss of labor due to morbidity (and eventual death), (2) time diverted to caring for the sick, and (3) loss of savings and assets in order to cope with disease and its impacts.

- **Labor:** Given the labor-intensive nature of agricultural systems in developing countries, disease and the associated loss of labor can have significant consequences. When illness leads to extended incapacitation or death of a productive household member, area cultivated and crop variety may decline. Cropping patterns may also change from more labor-intensive systems to less intensive ones.

FIg u r e 1   **Agriculture value-added per farmworker by income group, 2000 and 2005**

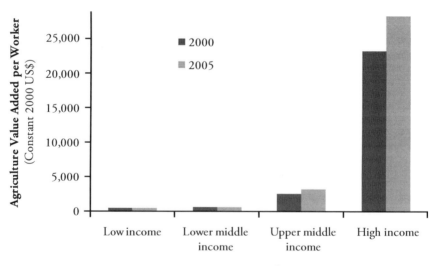

Source: World Bank 2008.

Healthy household members might also contribute to labor losses (and, thereby, productivity losses) because they must divert their time and energy from the farm to either take care of the sick family member or mourn and attend to burial or funeral matters.

- **Time:** The task of taking care of the sick typically falls to the women and girls of developing-country households, placing a burden on their already limited time. The amount of time diverted to caregiving, particularly for those with chronic or terminal illnesses, has implications for not only farm labor—since women typically do most labor-intensive farming activities like planting, weeding, and harvesting, particularly in Africa and especially for food production—but also to the viability of rural households overall. Household tasks—including fetching water and firewood, preparing food, cooking, cleaning, and caring for children—are time consuming and must be compromised or sacrificed entirely when a member of the family falls ill.

- **Assets:** The cost of healthcare is often prohibitive for farm families in developing countries. Households may need to respond to a family member's illness by the withdrawal of savings, selling important assets (such as jewelry, textiles, breeding animals, farm equipment, and land), withdrawing children from school, or reducing the nutritional value of their food consumption. All of these responses can have adverse effects on the labor productivity and overall well-being of household members.

Long-Term Impacts: r educed Productivity and Diminished Livelihood

A household's productivity depends on its health. In addition to the loss of household labor, health problems lower productivity in several other ways. Illness impairs the farmer's ability to innovate, experiment, and implement technical changes. Healthcare expenses may consume resources that otherwise might be used to purchase improved seed, fertilizer, equipment, or other inputs. And households with sick family members are less able to adopt labor-intensive techniques. Thus, the long-term household impacts of ill health include loss of farming knowledge, reduction of land under cultivation, planting of less labor-intensive crops, reduction of variety of crops planted, and reduction of livestock. Finally, the burden of high medical costs can trigger a chain reaction: reduced household food consumption may result in malnutrition that leads to diminished productivity and, ultimately, reduced resistance to disease.

Impacts of Farm Labor on Health

Just as health and disease can affect farm labor and productivity, the opposite is also true. Under ideal conditions, agriculture provides farmers and farm laborers with food, nutrition, and the income necessary to access water, land, information, education, and healthcare services.

But farm labor can also have an adverse effect on health and nutritional status due to the high expenditure of energy and time it demands—time that might be better spent on child care, food preparation, and nutrition-related activities. Farm labor can also expose workers to a range of occupational health hazards, such as accidents, diseases, and poisoning from pesticides. Farm labor can affect the health of workers through the following pathways.

- **Pesticide use:** As pesticide use has increased in developing countries, so, too, has pesticide poisoning in farmers, which can lead to hormone disruption; immune suppression; skin and eye damage; and chronic cardiopulmonary, neurological, and hematological problems. A recent estimate by the World Bank puts deaths caused by pesticide poisoning at 355,000 annually; two-thirds of those deaths occur in developing countries. Farm laborers do not always use protective clothing or equipment, which could be because (1) they are not aware of the dangers posed by pesticide exposure, (2) the necessary clothing and equipment are unavailable or unaffordable, or (3) there are no regulations enforcing these precautions. Many of the direct consequences from pesticides can be mitigated if protective measures are taken and recommended methods are followed when mixing and applying chemicals. Pesticides, however, also contaminate drinking water and crops that receive higher doses of pesticides, such as fruits and vegetables, thus posing serious health hazards to general consumers as well. Efforts to curtail this contamination will also require research, regulations, and monitoring.

  Improper use of pesticides also has less direct impacts on the health of farm laborers' family members and their overall household well-being. Research on a potato farming community in Ecuador revealed a rate of 171 pesticide poisonings per 100,000 people during 1991–92, which is 10 times the level reported by the Ministry of Health. Recuperation time averaged 11 days of lost labor wages, with the median indirect cost to the worker estimated at US$8.33 per case—more than five days' income (at US$1.50 per day). In addition to the main pesticide applicators, hospital records showed numerous cases of pesticide poisoning of women and children (Antle, Cole, and Crissman 1998). It is important to consider health effects in the economic analysis of pesticide adoption because the costs of crop loss to pests might well be lower than the direct (treatment) and indirect (lost income during recovery) costs of pesticide-related illness and the subsequent loss in farm labor productivity (Rola and Pingali 1993).

- **Labor migration:** Farm laborers are often migrant workers, due to the seasonal nature of agricultural production and the need for alternative income during off-peak seasons. Labor migration has implications for the spread of, and exposure to, various diseases. During the long dry season in the Sahel region of West Africa, for example, people migrate to the cocoa-growing areas to find jobs as farm laborers and take their earnings back to invest in farming ventures at home. This migration of people includes women who provide sexual services to the migrants. Any diseases, especially sexually transmitted diseases, contracted by farm laborers can then spread to migrants' household members in their areas of origin. In this respect, farm labor practices can have far-reaching negative effects on health and, in turn, work performance, productivity, and income (Hawkes and Ruel 2006a, 2006b).

- **Child labor:** When the availability of adult farm laborers is not sufficient to meet production needs, children may be taken out of school (if applicable) and made to work. All child labor, as defined by various organizations and governments, is, by its very nature, harmful and hazardous to a child's health, safety, and development.

- **Farm labor practices:** Certain practices and techniques employed by farm laborers can have inadvertent negative consequences on human and animal health. For example, crop rotation, irrigation, and the presence of livestock can create conditions that increase farm laborers' risk of contracting water-borne vector diseases (World Bank 2007). Similarly, some practices used to dry, store, and preserve maize, groundnuts, and other crops in regions with high levels of aflatoxins (naturally occurring toxic fungi that play a role in numerous infectious diseases) do little to prevent—and, in some cases, even increase—the spread of contamination. In these ways, the health of farm laborers and others can be sacrificed for the sake of productivity.

Policy r ecommendations

1. *Combat health threats to farm laborers through widespread education campaigns.* Among other locally specific concerns, these campaigns should include explanations of (1) the use of protective clothing to avoid the harmful effects of pesticides and (2) the danger of aflatoxins, their sources, and the proper food-commodity drying practices to avoid contamination. A long-term goal would be to enact legislation that enforces the safe use of pesticides and regulates testing, production, formulation, transportation, marketing, and disposal of pesticides in compliance with international standards.

2. *Design intervention activities that directly address the potential consequences of health and farm labor interactions.* Discussions between agriculture and health policymakers and professionals can help to identify and assess the externalities of projects—such as the disease-breeding conditions caused by some irrigation and water-storage techniques—and minimize their negative impacts.

3. *Enhance "win–win" practices that both increase farm labor productivity and improve nutrition.* With well-designed strategies—including home gardening, conservation farming, and cultivating aquaculture—rural farming households can make the most of their available labor resources.

4. *Collaborate more broadly through cross-sectoral, regional, and global programs.* Synergistic rural development calls for intersectoral partnerships between labor, agriculture, and health. Such partnerships will require regular monitoring and occasional impact assessments to assess effectiveness. Programs to combat animal disease, which is directly tied to human health (as evidenced by the spread of zoonotic and pandemic diseases) can also benefit from regional and global cooperation in surveillance, diagnosis, and treatment.

5. *Invest in essential research.* More information is needed on disease-specific impacts on farm labor productivity, including methodologies to measure farm labor productivity at the household level given the burden of disease. Studies should also be conducted on the potential impact of biofortified foods on nutrition and health. Promising pilot projects need to be adapted for broad applicability.

Concluding r emarks

Farm labor, agricultural productivity, and health are mutually interdependent; cumulatively, the health and the productivity of rural households determine the health of the agricultural sector. Research on mitigating the health threats to farm laborers in agricultural communities is essential to promoting regional and global development, reducing the incidence of disease, strengthening households' ability to cope with the effects of ill health, and mitigating its impacts on productivity.

r eferences

Antle, J. M., D. C. Cole, and C. C. Crissman. 1998. "Further Evidence on Pesticides, Productivity and Farmer Health: Potato Production in Ecuador." *Agricultural Economics* 18: 199–207.

Hawkes, C., and M. T. Ruel. 2006a. "The Links between Agriculture and Health: An Intersectoral Opportunity to Improve the Health and Livelihoods of the Poor." *Bulletin of the World Health Organization* 84 (12): 985–91.

———. 2006b. "Overview." In *Understanding the Links between Agriculture and Health.* edited by C. Hawkes and M. T. Ruel. 2020 Vision Focus 13, no. 1. Washington, DC: International Food Policy Research Institute.

Ravallion, M., S. Chen, and P. Sangraula. 2007. *New Evidence on the Urbanization of Global Poverty.* Policy Research Working Paper 4199. Washington, DC: World Bank.

Rola, A. C., and P. L. Pingali. 1993. *Pesticides, Rice Productivity, and Farmers' Health: An Economic Assessment.* Los Baños, Laguna, Philippines: World Resources Institute and International Rice Research Institute.

World Bank. 2008. *World Development Indicators.* Washington, DC.

Chapter 15

Addressing the Links among Agriculture, Malaria, and Development in Africa

Kwadwo Asenso-Okyere, Felix A. Asante, Jifar Tarekegn, and Kwaw S. Andam

The global impact of malaria on human health, productivity, and general well-being is profound, and Africa has been particularly hard hit. In 2006, more than 90 percent of deaths from malaria occurred in Africa, where 45 of the 53 countries are endemic for the disease (WHO 2008). Malaria costs Africa more than US$12 billion annually, and it slows economic growth in African countries by as much as 1.3 percent per year (WHO 2010).

Children and women (particularly pregnant women) in Africa are most vulnerable to malaria attacks. The potential impact of malaria for women engaged in agriculture, especially food production, can be substantial. Women perform nearly all the tasks associated with subsistence food production in Africa. They account for about 70 percent of agricultural workers and 60 to 80 percent of those producing foodcrops for household consumption and sale, and they also raise and market livestock (Todaro 2000; FAO 2010). Since the majority of the continent's population is rural, the effects of the disease on agriculture, health, and development are widespread.

Poor, rural farmers can pay quite a high cost for preventive measures and treatment. In Kenya and Nigeria, for example, estimates show annual treatment costs for small-scale farmers as high as 5 percent and 13 percent, respectively, of total household expenditure (WHO 1996). The burden is similar in other countries. To emphasize: *this is the cost borne by a household of poor smallholder farmers for treatment of a single disease.* Removing malaria as a constraint could free resources for household productivity and local development.

While most people can readily grasp the disease's impact on smallholder productivity and development, the impact of agriculture development on the disease is

This brief is based on the authors' IFPRI Discussion Paper (861) *The Linkages between Agriculture and Malaria: Issues for Policy, Research, and Capacity Strengthening* (Washington, DC: International Food Policy Research Institute, 2009).

less understood. Many agricultural practices increase the spread of malaria; in order to truly combat the disease, the risks involved in these practices must be managed and effective policy initiatives must take into account the two-way linkages between malaria and agricultural development.

The Impact of Malaria on Agricultural Development

Malaria's effects on smallholders can spiral. Taken ill at planting season, a farmer may not be able to cultivate as much land and engage in intensive farming practices. She may then plant less labor-intensive crops and change cropping patterns, perhaps raising crops with a lower return, and fewer of them. New techniques may be ignored because they require time and energy to learn, and the farmer may reduce inputs that require more energy or more money than the household has. The same may result if the farmer must take time off to care for her ill family members or if illness strikes at harvest time. Less land under cultivation, less effective methods, and a smaller harvest generate less income to pay for prevention and treatment (see Figure 1). Farm households may also withdraw savings, sell productive assets, or borrow money to pay for treatments. Fewer improvements may be made to farms, further decreasing their productivity even when illness is not an issue.

A recent United Nations report observed that "a brief period of illness that delays planting or coincides with the harvest may result in catastrophic economic effects" (UN Millennium Project 2005). Malaria transmission generally coincides with the planting and harvesting seasons, making the illness's impact particularly damaging.

Effects of Agricultural Development on Malaria

Farmers, communities, and programs may inadvertently be sowing seeds of their own ill health. Water resource development, deforestation, wetland cultivation, crop cover, land-use changes for agricultural purposes in the highlands, and an increase in urban agriculture all expand habitats for malaria-carrying mosquitoes. These practices, however, can also boost the income of producers, expanding access to preventive and treatment services and therefore improving health and productivity. The risks must be acknowledged and managed.

- **Water use and irrigation:** In Africa, irrigation exposes non-immune populations in areas of unstable malaria transmission to a high risk of acquiring the disease. This effect of irrigation—creating conditions for the transmission of malaria—may be one of the most severe negative consequences of water projects.

- **Deforestation:** While deforestation can reduce the breeding habitats of mosquitoes that breed in shaded water, changes in environmental and climatic conditions in the deforested region can also promote the survival of other species, leading to prolonged seasons of malaria transmission.

- **Wetlands:** The cultivation of valley bottoms across East Africa as a result of population growth and demand for food has changed the local ecology. These wetlands were covered with natural papyrus, which limits the breeding of the *Anopheles gambiae* mosquito because of the denseness of the vegetation and the natural oil layer. The elimination of the papyrus and the reclamation of the swamps have led to an increase in temperatures, which promotes the breeding and survival of mosquitoes and increases malaria transmission (WHO 2008).

- **Crop cover:** Thickets formed by crop cover could be favorable environments for mosquito breeding, although to date there is little documented evidence. It may be possible for mosquitoes to breed in leaf axils (for example, of pineapples, bananas, cocoyams, and maize), tree holes, and bamboo stumps. It is known that maize pollen provides nutrition for larval carrier mosquitoes.

FIgu r E 1   Conceptual framework for the impact of malaria on agriculture

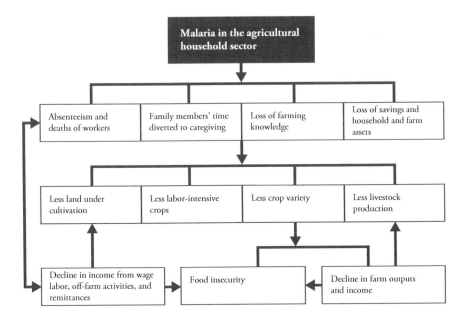

Source: Negin 2004, with authors' modifications.

- **Highlands:** The increasing incidence of malaria in the highlands, especially in Eastern Africa, has been attributed largely to agricultural practices that have changed rainfall patterns, temperature, and vegetation. The reemergence of malaria in the highlands of western Kenya has been blamed on forest clearing for the development of tea estates and the migration of labor to the farms. The construction of access roads through the forests to the farms, the building of milldams on rivers, and the massive deforestation, among other factors, have caused a drastic change in the ecology, making it suitable for the breeding of malaria-carrying mosquitoes. Similar observations have been made in the Amani hills of Tanzania, the Rukungiri and Kabale districts of southwest Uganda, and the Rwanda highlands.

- **Urban agriculture:** It is generally held that malaria in Africa is predominantly a rural disease and that mosquito breeding decreases with urbanization. However, in some African cities, poor environmental management and peri-urban agriculture provide favorable habitats for mosquitoes.

Blending Effective Agricultural, Health, and Development Policies

Since the majority of the world's and Africa's poor, work in agriculture and the poor suffer disproportionately from related illness and disease, an integrated view of agriculture, development, and health is necessary to promote agricultural growth, reduce pervasive rural poverty, and improve well-being.

- *Tackle the threat of malaria at the start of agricultural water development projects.* Water projects often support the breeding of mosquitoes, and the density of the malarial mosquito population often indicates transmission rates. This is not true in all cases, however. With sufficient preventive care and mosquito control, not only can downward spirals of health and productivity be avoided but the people can also be productive enough to purchase adequate treatment on their own and begin an upward surge of development. Water projects should therefore include provisions for effective vector control, effective water management, and prevention interventions.

- *Coordinate health and agriculture policy efforts.* Even though the linkage between agriculture and health was first recognized long ago, health considerations still play little part in governments' agricultural policy decisions. The health sector also has not reached out to agriculture as a key partner in addressing global ill health.

Because malaria and agricultural development have a well-integrated relationship, integrated policies are best suited to address them.

- *Aggressively disseminate information about the two-way interaction between malaria and agriculture.* While most rural populations are aware of malaria as a serious illness and recognize the link between mosquitoes and the disease, fewer people understand the linkage between malaria and agriculture in terms of causation and impact. Information about the linkages, prevention practices, and treatments aimed at farmers and extension workers could lead to capacity-building activities. It should be an essential part of all rural agriculture and health projects. Similar information should accompany farm inputs (seeds, tools, fertilizers, and so forth) at purchase. Information should be geared particularly toward women, as they are often the primary agricultural producers.

- *Intensify public health interventions just before and during the growing season.* Researchers have noted that bouts of malaria particularly threaten livelihoods when they occur in the planting, growing, and harvesting seasons and that this is when they are most likely to occur. Effective timing of interventions (inoculations, clinic openings, information campaigns, and so forth) is thus crucial and likely to pay the greatest dividends.

- *Conduct research to target interventions even further.* Although information on malaria's effects on agricultural productivity exists, it is inadequate due to the nature of the disease and the coping mechanisms that families adopt. Research can shed light on malaria's direct negative effects on farm households' food security, nutrition, and livelihood and could lead to more focused policy.

Concluding remarks

There is widespread recognition among African leaders, international organizations, and the donor community that improving agriculture's productivity and income-generating capacity is essential to poverty reduction and economic growth. This means that malaria must be addressed. The disease's impact on the agricultural sector is widely felt in Africa since about 70 percent of Africa's population engages in agriculture. Ill health from malaria causes a decline in crop output, a reduction in the use of inputs, a decrease in area planted, changes in cropping patterns, and loss of agricultural knowledge. Unfortunately, agricultural practices and projects can increase the spread of malaria. Efforts to address the disease and improve agricultural development must take this two-way relationship into account.

r eferences

FAO (Food and Agriculture Organization of the United Nations). 2010. "Towards Sustainable Food Security: Women and Sustainable Food Security." Accessed December 2, www.fao.org/sd/fsdirect/fbdirect/FSP001.htm.

Negin, J. 2004. "Impact of HIV/AIDS on Agriculture," in *The Impact of AIDS,* edited by United Nations Secretariat, Population Division. New York: United Nations.

Todaro, M. P. 2000. *Economic Development,* 7th ed. New York: Addison-Wesley Longman.

UN Millennium Project. 2005. *Coming to Grips with Malaria in the New Millennium.* Task Force on HIV/AIDS, Malaria, TB, and Access to Essential Medicines, Working Group on Malaria. London and Sterling, VA, US: Earthscan.

WHO (World Health Organization). 1996. "Effects of Agriculture and Vector-Borne Diseases." In *Agricultural Development and Vector-Borne Diseases: Training and Information Materials on Vector Biology and Control in the VBC Slide Set Series.* Geneva: WHO/FAO/UNEP/UNCHS Panel of Experts on Environmental Management for Vector Control [PEEM] Secretariat.

————. 2008. *World Malaria Report.* Geneva: WHO.

————. 2010. "Economic Costs of Malaria." 2001–2010 United Nations Decade to Roll Back Malaria. Accessed December 2, http://rbm.who.int/cmc_upload/0/000/015/363/RBMInfosheet_10.htm.

Chapter 16

Gender: A Key Dimension Linking Agricultural Programs to Improved Nutrition and Health

Ruth Meinzen-Dick, Julia Behrman, Purnima Menon, and Agnes Quisumbing

I mproving the livelihoods and well-being of the rural poor is an important aim of agricultural development. But improved agricultural productivity does not necessarily translate into improved health and nutrition, either for producers or consumers. How can standard agricultural development strategies—promoting agricultural intensification, greater linkages to markets, and high-value production—also create positive impacts on health and nutrition? This chapter argues that a key element linking these programs to improved outcomes is the dimension of gender roles and gender equity.

A large body of evidence shows that, in many parts of the world, men and women spend money differently: women are more likely to spend the income they control on food, healthcare, and education of their children. Increasing household income does not necessarily improve the nutritional and health status of women and children when that income is controlled by men. Women's relative bargaining power within the household is likely to influence whether gains in income translate into nutritional improvements. Empirical evidence shows that increasing women's control over land, physical assets, and financial assets serves to raise agricultural productivity, improve child health and nutrition, and increase expenditures on education, contributing to overall poverty reduction (World Bank 2001; Quisumbing 2003).

Arimond and colleagues have identified five pathways through which agricultural interventions can affect nutrition: increased food for own consumption; increased income; reductions in market prices; shifts in preferences; and shifts in control of resources within households (2010). They highlight the substantial influence of gender roles across all five pathways, particularly in relation to increased food availability and increased income. A key gender-related factor that affects

This chapter is based on the authors' 2020 Conference Brief, *Gender: A Key Dimension Linking Agricultural Programs to Improved Nutrition and Health* (Washington, DC: International Food Policy Research Institute, 2011).

the impact of agricultural interventions on nutrition is whether the agricultural intervention enhances women's control over assets.

Three agricultural development strategies are discussed in this chapter, to illustrate the significance of the gender dimension in promoting improved nutrition and health: (1) linking smallholders to markets, (2) large-scale agriculture, and (3) homestead food production.

Linking Smallholders to Markets

Linking smallholders to high-value markets can increase their incomes while maintaining decentralized production arrangements. The two main approaches currently used in linking farmers to markets are *contract farming* and *producer marketing groups*. In contract farming, supermarkets, agroprocessors, or exporters offer to buy products from individual smallholders, often paying more than the local market price. The contractor may provide inputs and training to help smallholders deliver the quantity and quality needed for higher-value markets. Producer marketing groups, organized by outsiders or by farmers themselves, promote access to higher-value markets through shared transport or bulk contracts, or disseminating new farming practices among members.

Studies of the nutrition impacts of cash-cropping and commercialization, conducted in the 1990s, were instrumental in calling attention to the importance of gender and intrahousehold allocation for nutrition. The nutrition impact of programs that link smallholder farmers to markets has yet to be fully analyzed. Contract farming agreements that do not pay attention to intrahousehold labor allocation and decisionmaking may in fact aggravate the dynamics that disadvantage vulnerable household members.

- One large-scale venture in China contracted exclusively with the senior male members of each household, even though women did most of the agricultural work, leading to disputes because women were often not properly compensated for their work.

- In contrast, one example of contract farming for nontraditional export crops in the Dominican Republic increased the demand for women's farm labor, while also providing women an opportunity to demand compensation for their labor.

- Case studies of cotton contract farming in Zambia indicate that, with deliberate targeting of female participants and promotion of gender-friendly enterprises, contract farming can be profitable for female farmers.

Producer groups potentially offer farmers greater control in choosing crops and production methods, but it is essential, in working with such groups, to ascertain whether they represent both men and women. In working with groups dominated by men, more gender-equitable outcomes can be achieved either by increasing women's involvement in the farmers' associations or by working with separate male and female farmers' associations. The effectiveness of these approaches will depend on how comfortable women are with articulating their interests in the presence of men. In Zimbabwe, for example, women have developed their own Women Farmers' Union; while in Zambia, a woman leads the national dairy group and has become the first woman member of the national committee of the farmers' union.

A recurring problem for market-oriented smallholder strategies is to ensure that women maintain control of their income. In Kenyan tea production, women's bargaining power was greater in households where women's labor was indispensable than in households that relied on hired labor. Where women are less able to transport produce to market, men generally make the financial transactions and retain the income. When farming enterprises under female control become more profitable, they may be taken over by men, as occurred in Kenyan household milk production—to the detriment of household (and especially children's) nutrition.

Fortunately, new methods of payment make it easier to ensure that payments for women's production go directly to women. Women who are members of microfinance groups or producer groups (such as milk unions) can receive payments into their own accounts. Payment systems via mobile phones further expand the options for women to receive payments directly. Ensuring that women maintain control of production after it becomes profitable represents a greater challenge, however; effective approaches may involve working directly with men or providing them profitable business opportunities, so that increases in women's income are not seen as diminishing men's income.

Finally, access to so-called "higher-value markets" requires meeting certain standards for the final product. Compliance with such standards carries both risks and opportunities. Cash-constrained smallholders may cut corners on safety equipment or increase pesticide applications, creating health hazards that pose a greater threat to women, and particularly pregnant women. Compliance with important biosafety standards, such as control of aflatoxin exposure, may be more difficult for women producers, who have less access to information or the necessary cash for control measures. These obstacles reduce the marketability of their produce.

Gendered constraints to adoption of standards, including issues of communication and affordability, need to be addressed to ensure that these standards improve food safety without excluding women or poor producers. As recently recommended, gender-focused analyses of value chains could substantially help in addressing such bottlenecks.[1] Enhancing women's control over production, income, and assets will make a significant contribution toward improving the nutrition and health impacts of agricultural development strategies that link smallholder farmers with markets.

Recommendations

The potential gender disparities of programs linking smallholders to markets need to be directly addressed to realize their full benefits for improved health and nutrition.

- Include women producers in contracts and group membership, and make payments directly to women.

- In commercializing food crops or expanding cash crops, ensure that control does not shift from women to men, compromising household food security.

- Integrate health and safety concerns with the introduction of new technologies and markets; ensure that both women and men are trained to minimize exposure to agrochemicals and ensure compliance with biosafety requirements.

Large-Scale Agriculture

The large-farm model is substantially different from family farming: ownership, management, and labor are often distinct roles; and production may be vertically integrated with processing, marketing, and export logistics. While research interest in plantations has recently increased, there has been limited research on either the nutrition impacts or the gender implications of large-scale agriculture (Behrman, Meinzen-Dick, and Quisumbing 2011).

This chapter identifies two primary pathways through which large-scale agriculture influences nutrition: (1) by increasing the income of agricultural workers; and (2) by affecting the level of control that women exercise over household income. Health and nutrition outcomes can also be affected by working conditions, healthcare, childcare, other facilities, and environmental impacts. Large-scale agriculture thus offers a range of opportunities for gender-equitable policies that reinforce health and nutrition.

Women's employment in large-scale farms depends in part on the type of crop and in part on other factors: the degree of mechanization, types of labor (formal or

---

1 For nutrition-focused analyses of value chains, see Corinna Hawkes and Marie Ruel, *Value Chains for Nutrition,* 2020 Conference Brief 4 (Washington, DC: International Food Policy Research Institute, 2011).

informal, permanent or temporary), compensation agreements, and the possibility of combining plantation work with other agricultural and domestic activities. While mechanized farming can limit employment opportunities for local populations, some research indicates that a system of partially mechanized production—increasingly prevalent in plantations in Africa—can be advantageous to women. In sugar cane production, for example, machines are used for cutting the cane, the most physically challenging job, reserved for men, but the workers gather it manually. This system can create more employment and more income for women.

Working conditions can substantially affect the health and nutrition of farm-based employees. Case studies in India find that women hired in wage labor systems often encounter lower wages and worse working conditions than men, along with difficulties in negotiating for better compensation or conditions. Women who are undercompensated and overworked are less able to fulfill their role as the household providers of health and nutrition. Provision of adequate childcare facilities is also important. Without childcare, women working as laborers are often forced to take their young children into the fields, a situation that can lead to child labor and expose young children to risks of zoonotic (animal-borne) disease, harmful pesticides, or work related injuries. Alternatively, mothers may leave young children in the care of older children, usually girls, with negative impacts on both the care of the children and the schooling of the older girls. Large-scale agricultural systems may in some cases be better able to provide healthcare, schooling, and childcare, benefiting women and children.

The use of pesticides and other agrochemicals in large-scale farms may have serious health effects on the men and women who work as wage laborers. Even more problematic is that laborers may track residue of pesticides back into their homes and expose children or other vulnerable family members to these agrochemicals. This is especially likely when workers do not have adequate training, safety gear, or cleaning facilities. Pregnant women are particularly vulnerable to agrochemical exposure.

Moreover, the "gendering" of tasks can lead to greater pesticide exposure for women, as in the following examples:

- A case study of biofuels plantations in Indonesia finds women are assigned the tasks of spraying and fertilizer application, and protective gear is available only at the worker's expense (Julia and White 2010).

- In the Latin American cut-flower industry, flower workers are exposed to a variety of harmful pesticides without adequate safeguards, leading to a higher than normal rate of miscarriage (Paz-y-Mino et al. 2002); women workers, who are paid on commission, spend more time in greenhouses than male workers, who possess formal contracts.

- A study from the International Labour Organization indicates that women workers in plantations often receive less training and instruction regarding the application of agrochemicals than male counterparts (Loewenson 2000).

Plantation systems may also have important *environmental impacts* with gender dimensions. Discharge of pollutants may damage the quality of local soil and water. The demand for water to sustain large-scale agricultural production will likely compete with water needed for food production, livestock, and domestic consumption. Women are typically responsible for collecting water and fuel, and may be forced to seek out less reliable and more distant sources. In addition, women often make use of wild-growing plant species for household consumption, and these varieties may be reduced by monoculture plantations. Although many of these environmental problems may also occur with other commercial monocropping systems, they are particularly problematic in plantations because of the scale of such systems, and the fact that those who make decisions about production may not be those most affected by the decisions.

In sum, the nutrition and health impacts of large farms and plantations are largely determined by their effect on household incomes of farm workers and by their environmental externalities, and these impacts affect women and men differently. While many case studies give cause for concern, fair trade and corporate social responsibility provide a basis for positive outcomes. A notable example is the fairtrade export of cut flowers from Kenya and Tanzania to Norway, which provides high levels of female-dominated employment, equal contracts for men and women (including maternity and paternity leave), safety standards, and social engagement.

Recommendations

Large-scale agricultural operations can avoid disadvantaging women and communities by being gender-aware as well as by observing environmental safeguards.

- Ensure that employment opportunities—including task allocation, hours worked, wages, and promotion possibilities—are gender equitable.

- Provide appropriate and affordable healthcare and childcare facilities.

- Ensure that new technologies—such as mechanization, new crops and varieties, inorganic fertilizer, and pesticides—are introduced in a gender-sensitive manner.

- Provide appropriate safety equipment and training to both female and male laborers.

• Minimize the negative environmental impacts of plantations on the local community.

Homestead Food Production

Homestead food production (HFP) has attracted attention as an agricultural development strategy, particularly for households with limited land. Linkages among gender, agriculture, health, and nutrition are easily traced: the strategy aims to increase dietary diversity using household labor intensively on small gardens within the homestead, allowing women to grow a variety of fruits and vegetables and tend small livestock while fulfilling their domestic and child care responsibilities.

Helen Keller International (HKI), an international nongovernmental organization (NGO), pioneered this model to address vitamin-A deficiency in Bangladesh in the 1980s. HKI expanded and adapted the program for Cambodia, Nepal, and the Philippines in the late 1990s, through strategic partnerships with more than 200 local nongovernmental and governmental organizations. The HFP model was broadened to include small animal husbandry in order to address multiple micronutrient deficiencies, including iron and zinc; the program in Cambodia included chicken and duck production in addition to vegetables. This aspect, too, is consistent with women's asset accumulation strategies: women tend to own and care for small livestock, while men are responsible for larger animals.

HFP programming has evolved to address other aspects of food insecurity, including improved incomes and livelihoods, community development, and the empowerment of women. Programs operate in several countries of South Asia, Southeast Asia and the Pacific, and Sub-Saharan Africa. A number of research studies and reviews of the nutrition impacts of HFP programs indicate that the effective HFP models take into account several gender-related factors: women's control over assets; nutrition education and behavior change communication about allocation of household resources to safeguard vulnerable household members, such as mothers and young children; and key messages regarding optimal infant and young-child feeding and care practices.

Gender norms differ across countries and contexts, so the appropriate means for addressing gender concerns will also differ. In Bangladesh, programs built on women's traditional role as providers of food and care within the household; at the same time, they addressed constraints on women's access to agricultural land and credit, as well as norms that favor social seclusion. Programs have used women's groups to introduce homestead vegetable production, creating income sources that women control. In the HKI Burkina Faso homestead food production program, project staff led preliminary communitywide sensitizations, to make men as well as women aware of the importance of maternal nutrition and improved maternal and child feeding practices—so that husbands would refrain from appropriating the produce or proceeds of women's gardens.

To be sustainable, HFP programs must generate income over the long run. This may require diversifying income sources—such as through small livestock—and improving links to markets. In Bangladesh, one NGO introduced new vegetable technologies, and then helped establish marketing channels in Dhaka for the produce. Another focused on homestead milk production, hiring female livestock workers and modifying bicycles so women could use them to collect milk. Moving the focus of the dairy value chain from the market to the homestead helped increase women's participation, and linked the homestead to the market.

Recommendations

Taking gender roles into account can help HFP programs improve health and nutrition. The following are key strategies:

- Encourage diversified gardens that include high-value crops and small livestock in order to increase dietary diversity, provide sources of additional income, and enable women to accumulate assets.

- Explicitly address nutrition education and behavior change and communication in HFP programs.

- Identify gender-specific constraints on participation.

- Foster income generation and better links to markets.

Conclusions and Policy Implications

There is substantial evidence confirming the impact on health and nutritional outcomes of strengthening the position of women, both in terms of control of resources and agricultural productivity, and in terms of relative bargaining power within the household. However, research is needed to fully understand the linkages between alternative agricultural development strategies on health and nutrition. Just as gender relations are culture and context specific, the appropriate agricultural development strategy will vary both across and within countries.

As agricultural productivity increases and surplus food is marketed, the distinction between food and cash crops at the household level will tend to erode. Two areas are likely to be of concern: (1) at the national or aggregate level, the balance between food and cash crops, as biofuels (for example) and food crops compete for scarce farmland; and (2) at the household level, the control over income derived from various crops.

Homestead food production is still an underutilized strategy. Combined with educational and other initiatives, it potentially offers substantial improvements in health and nutrition. Evidence indicates that even small-scale homestead production of micronutrient-rich foods, when combined with nutrition education, can have impact greater than its income effects. Homestead production systems offer the potential to improve nutrition for peri-urban and agricultural laborer households, as well as small farmers.

In any production or employment scenario, however, the available evidence indicates that increasing women's access to resources and control over household income will have important implications for the health and nutrition of the family, and particularly of women and children.

From the perspective of nutrition and some aspects of health, therefore, any development strategy should explicitly consider its impacts on women and children—and especially on the critical "window of opportunity" from preconception through the second year of life, when nutritional deprivation and toxic environmental exposures can have lifelong consequences. In designing agricultural development projects, planners must make informed provisions for

- reducing environmental toxin risks;

- providing optimal childcare, either through maternity leave policies or through provision of adequate childcare facilities;

- ensuring that women have adequate control over income, resources, and time; and

- providing nutrition and health education—ideally, simultaneous with agricultural interventions.

For researchers in this field, the urgent priority is to develop further evidence on the full impacts of various forms of agricultural development, both on women's control over income and assets, and on health and nutrition. The development impact of agricultural investments cannot be understood without considering their nutritional, health, and gender-based effects.

References

Arimond, M., C. Hawkes, M. T. Ruel, Z. Sifri, P. R. Berti, J. L. Leroy, J. W. Low, L. R. Brown, and E. A. Frongillo. 2010. "Agricultural Interventions and Nutrition: Lessons from the Past and New Evidence." In *Combating Micronutrient Deficiencies: Food-Based Approaches,* edited by B. Thompson and L. Amoroso. Rome: Food and Agriculture Organization of the United Nations and CAB International.

Behrman, J., R. Meinzen-Dick, and A. Quisumbing. 2011. *Gender Implications of Large Scale Land Deals.* IFPRI Discussion Paper. Washington DC: International Food Policy Research Institute.

Loewenson, R. 2000. "Occupational Safety and Health for Women Workers in Agriculture." *Labour Education* 1–2 (118–119): 35–45.

Paz-y-Mino C., G. Bustamante, M. E. Sanchez, and P. E. Leone. 2002. "Cytogenetic Monitoring in a Population Occupationally Exposed to Pesticides in Ecuador." *Environmental Health Perspectives* 110 (11): 1077–80.

Quisumbing, Agnes R., ed. 2003. *Household Decisions, Gender, and Development: A Synthesis of Recent Research.* Washington, DC: International Food Policy Research Institute.

World Bank. 2001. *Engendering Development: Gender Equality in Rights, Resources, and Voice.* New York: Oxford University Press for the World Bank.

Chapter 17

Cross-Sectoral Coordination in the Public Sector: A Challenge to Leveraging Agriculture for Improving Nutrition and Health

Todd Benson

ood nutrition and health for all are recognized as socially desirable objectives around the globe. It is generally accepted that national and local governments have a duty to provide the goods and services necessary for maintaining good nutrition and health. Moreover, improved health and nutrition are critical inputs for achieving broad economic growth and poverty reduction.

Malnutrition and ill health arise from a combination of causes and thus require efforts across multiple sectors to address them effectively. The *health* and *agriculture* sectors are central to such efforts, reflecting their mandates to provide curative and preventative health services and to facilitate food production. However, several other sectors must contribute their efforts as well: the *education* sector, given the importance of knowledge to proper nutrition and healthcare practices; the *water, sanitation,* and *housing* sectors to promote hygienic environments; the *labor* sector to maintain adequate household incomes; and *public finance* and *planning* agencies to ensure that government resources are appropriately allocated.

In short, healthy and active lives for all require adequate access to food, care, employment, health services, and a healthy environment. None of these determinants of good health and nutrition is sufficient by itself; all of them are necessary. The most efficient policy approach involves, accordingly, a coordinated effort across the various public sector ministries and agencies concerned. However, most governments and government agencies are organized in a way that makes coordination across sectors difficult to achieve.

This chapter considers how these organizational barriers might be overcome, particularly in relation to the public agriculture sector. We examine the structure,

This chapter is extracted from the author's IFPRI Research Report (156), *Improving Nutrition as a Development Priority: Addressing Undernutrition within National Policy Processes in Sub-Saharan Africa* (Washington, DC: International Food Policy Research Institute, 2008).

priorities, and core competencies of sectoral agencies in government. Based on this overview, several approaches are suggested to foster better collaboration between agriculture and other sectors of government.

Organizational Barriers to Cross-Sectoral Action

Government bureaucracies have emerged as a generally successful solution to the problem of managing the activities of states. Ideally, they are organized on the basis of clear goals, rational functional specialization of sub-units, formal operating procedures, and clear lines of authority. Most governments are organized administratively within a framework of sectoral agencies, including separate ministries for health, education, agriculture, and other sectors. Political and administrative power is exercised within this framework, and resource allocations, incentives, and systems of accountability are managed accordingly.

However, most bureaucracies are not organized in a manner that facilitates broad, effective efforts to address a problem requiring actions across sectors. So, even though achieving good health and nutrition for all might be government's responsibility, the sectoral organization of the public bureaucracy clearly hinders undertaking the necessary joint action.

There are three overlapping barriers to effective joint action across government sectors: (1) the differing worldviews and mandates of sectors; (2) the resource allocation and planning processes within government; and (3) capacity constraints within sectors for generating necessary information.

Sectoral Worldviews

The specialized training of various sector specialists tends to lead to discrete areas of expertise and qualitatively different worldviews. In considering a development problem, experts tend to embrace information within their own discipline while disregarding other matters as irrelevant to taking action on the issue. Agriculture sector objectives, for example, relate principally to increasing yields, profits, and other benefits for producers, and they are reflected in distinctive language and methods. Health and nutrition considerations do not fit neatly into the worldview of agriculture or the sector's mandates.

Moreover, the expertise of sectoral specialists is applied within the context of formally stated mandates and objectives, which distinguish areas of institutional specialization within the government bureaucracy as a whole and define expected courses of action. These sectoral priorities are an important element in planning processes, as they are the basis by which an institution within a sector can make substantive claims on state resources. Likewise, for civil servants, personal incentives like career advancement will be linked to their contribution to the attainment of these narrowly defined objectives of the sector within which they work, rather than broader objectives requiring joint action with other sectors. Cross-sectoral efforts to improve nutrition and health also face the problem of funding, as these issues do not represent a priority area of focus for any of the sectors involved. Agriculturalists, for example, can be expected to allocate any resources put at their disposal toward addressing their core mandate of increasing agricultural productivity—rather than devoting resources to secondary issues requiring coordinated action with other sectors.

Competing for Resources across Sectors
In general, the resource allocation processes of government budgeting and human-resource management make it difficult to mount cross-sectoral action. Each sector must compete with other sectors for the resources it requires. Typically, budgeting is viewed as a zero-sum game by sector managers: funding that goes to another sector, even if for coordinated cross-sectoral activities, is viewed as a loss of resources for their own sector.

Similarly, sector-specific criteria form the basis for evaluating sector effectiveness and hence for the allocation of resources. The resource allocation mechanisms provide limited, if any, incentives for carrying out joint coordinated activities, even though they may potentially have greater impact on broader development priorities. The attainment of objectives requiring cross-sectoral, coordinated action will rarely be advanced by routine sector-planning mechanisms.

Limited Information for Action
Specialists within each sector, including agriculture, often lack the expertise needed to recognize either the determinants of ill health and poor nutritional status or effective approaches to addressing these problems. Greater capacity for analysis of these kinds of cross-cutting development challenges would increase sectoral leaders' understanding of the synergies that can be attained by concerted effort. However, it seems unlikely that, in the course of normal operations, sectors will try to build expertise on issues outside their own sphere.

In sum, there are substantial institutional and operational barriers in most countries that prevent the agriculture sector from accepting a share of responsibility for the problems of ill-health and malnutrition in society. Many of these barriers are simply a reflection of a rational sectoral organization that enables government to fulfill many of its duties. In general, the goal of sustainably addressing the challenges of health and nutrition fit poorly within a bureaucratic organization and its operational processes and incentive structures.

Political Context

Advocacy is essential to foster the agriculture sector's increased attention on issues related to improved health and nutrition. The form that effective advocacy takes will depend on both the particular issue and the specific context of policy and resource allocation decisions.

"Pressing" versus "Chosen" Policy Issues

Grindle and Thomas usefully distinguish between *pressing* and *chosen* policy problems (1989). When a policy concern is pressing, substantive policy reform and action to address the issue is more likely to occur than when the concern is viewed as optional — or, "politics-as-usual" — and policymakers can choose not to address it without incurring political risk. Most of the issues related to improved health and nutrition that involve agriculture tend to fall into the politics-as-usual category. Ill health and malnutrition may be widely viewed as primarily a responsibility of the household and not of the government. Similarly, poor health, high morbidity, and food insecurity may be considered part of the environment within which a government operates, rather than as public issues to be addressed. In most developing countries, the effectiveness and legitimacy of political leaders are unlikely to be called into question because of, say, continuing rates of high infant mortality or prevalence of stunted children. Unfortunately, these are treated as political issues of choice rather than urgency.

Alternative perspectives on a health or nutrition problem can, however, reframe an issue and sharpen public perception of its urgency. Through creative advocacy, a broad understanding can be crafted that could call into question a government's legitimacy based on its attention to health and nutrition issues. The framing and definition of the policy issue is critical to determining its characterization.

Drivers of Policy Formulation

The structures and mechanisms through which a government establishes its priorities vary considerably across countries. In many countries, political parties and special interest groups engage in the policy process, contributing to its dynamism — both defining the problems to be addressed and suggesting solutions for them. Within a democratic context, the actual decisionmaking structures are primarily those instituted to enable decisions by citizen representatives — that is, legislatures and cabinets; while government institutions are primarily only responsible for implementation of the resulting policies. The overall process exemplifies what Grindle and Thomas have called *society-centered* policy processes.

In contrast, in many developing countries, democratic institutions at the national level are absent or relatively new; there is less scope for a representative electoral system to influence problem definition and agenda-setting in policy debates. Often, most of the relevant expertise on a particular policy issue is found within government. In nations characterized by such *state-centered* policy processes, government institutions tend to play a significantly larger role in driving policy-making than they do in countries with society-centered policy processes.

Effective forms of advocacy will differ depending on the nature of a country's policy processes. Where society-centered processes dominate, engagement with broad civil society and political organizations will be an important component of any advocacy strategy. However, the greatest burdens of ill health and malnutrition are found in countries where state-centered policy processes dominate. In those cases, much of the advocacy effort needs to focus principally on engaging political leaders and the technocratic elites of government. These state-actors have great leeway to set government priorities and control the allocation of its resources.

Creating Openings for Agriculture to Contribute to Better Nutrition and Health

Three approaches have been used to overcome barriers to cross-sectoral action: policy champions, civil society coalitions, and community-based efforts.

Policy Champions

The state-centered nature of policymaking in many target countries, as well as the need for cross-sectoral policy responses, makes individual leadership critical in addressing ill health and malnutrition. But because efforts to improve health and nutrition do not fit neatly into sectoral programming, the institutional organization of government does not by itself produce institutional champions of, or advocates for, these issues at the highest levels (Benson 2007). Within national policy processes, the leaders of formal government institutions are not expected to take on responsibility for ensuring that sufficient state resources are allocated to addressing ill health and malnutrition or for addressing the multiple determinants of these problems. Without such leadership, and given limited resources and human capacity, the routine operations of government are unlikely to lead to effective public efforts to improve health and nutrition.

Because politicians and other members of the policy elite are unlikely to automatically increase the resources allocated to activities that improve health and nutrition, the motivation to do so must come from outside the formal organization and processes of government. A key advocacy strategy is to cultivate policy champions as the visible leaders of campaigns to include health and nutrition among the priorities of the government and its sectoral bodies. These champions need to be properly informed on the issues, well connected, and persistent, and they need to have access to the various venues for policy debates. These traits are more important than having technical qualifications on the issues they champion.

Civil Society Advocacy Coalitions

The activities of champions of health and nutrition issues need to be coordinated with any technical efforts being promoted on these issues, to ensure that their policy influence is adequately informed. Given the problems of establishing leadership within government on cross-sectoral efforts to bring about sustained improvements in health and nutrition, there is considerable merit in the formation of a national advocacy coalition around these issues to foster such action. Such coalitions should include individuals from civil society, international agencies, and private institutions, as well as government, who are committed to achieving good health and nutrition for all, both as a human right and as a basis for human and economic development. The members of the advocacy coalition should work in a coordinated fashion to focus government attention on these issues and to increase the level of public resources allocated to address them.

Such a national civil society advocacy group may be essential to make substantive progress on these issues that are not adequately addressed in sectoral agendas, as a way of bringing agriculture and other relevant sectors into action on health and nutrition. However, given the difficulty of establishing policy leadership on broad health and nutrition issues, the creation of such coalitions is problematic. Leadership and participation in such advocacy efforts will often depend on chance: the personal qualities of individuals—their training, experience, personal values, and vision—may prompt them to become involved. Nevertheless, such a process can also be seeded. Topical health and nutrition concerns that involve agricultural issues, such as the formulation of national food security and nutrition strategies, can often provide a kernel group of nutrition advocates, whose membership, functions, and areas of focus can then be expanded.

Community and Other Decentralized Efforts

Community-directed efforts can also provide important incentives for agriculturalists to contribute to efforts to improve health and nutrition, working in concert with other sectors. Community development needs rarely fit neatly into particular sectoral competencies, but rather require contributions from multiple sectors. Community demand for government assistance in addressing a problem thus provides an immediate incentive for cross-sectoral action. Where governments are strongly committed to supporting community-driven efforts, adequate leadership for cross-sectoral activities may flourish in spite of the bureaucratic organization of the sectors. Moreover, the resource conflicts between sectors typically play out at the national level; at more local levels, civil servants may have limited control over sector resource allocations, so the stakes between sectors are lower.

However, the ability of state agencies to work collaboratively, even in assisting communities, will vary widely. In Ghana and Uganda, government decentralization has progressed further than in most countries, but even in those countries district-level agriculturalists stated that local concerns were not necessarily more important than sectoral concerns in guiding their actions (Benson 2008). These agriculturalists were still subordinate to sectoral superiors, they operated with limited resources, and many of the incentives for individual effort served to hamper cross-sectoral action to assist communities. Thus, while community-directed development *may* promote increased attention from agriculturalists to local health and nutrition problems, it is not guaranteed.

Conclusion

The institutional barriers faced by public sector agriculturalists trying to improve health and nutrition are durable and strong. Consequently, an opportunistic approach may be more effective in practice than strong, programmatic action by the sector or even by several sectors. An opportunistic strategy would piggyback on existing individual activities in the agricultural sector or other sectors in an instrumental way, to address important context-specific determinants of ill-health and malnutrition. Working in this incremental manner appears more likely to be successful than mounting a large-scale, cross-sectoral implementation effort that is a poor fit within the institutional framework of government. Such a task- or problem-oriented approach would start small, achieve short-term goals, and build on these successes iteratively to address larger problems. Individual sectoral responses will often be the best that can be realistically expected.

Consequently, one should be cautious of launching any health or nutrition program that depends on intersectoral coordination. The risk is too great that such coordination will not happen. However, an important first step is simply to ensure that the agriculture sector (or any other relevant sector) takes seriously its potential role in improving health and nutrition. Cross-sectoral coordination emerges as a practical issue once the problems of health and nutrition are treated as politically important, stimulating leadership for action on the problems in various sectors. Coordinated efforts should follow, once such commitments are clear.

Health and nutrition can be improved through agricultural means. There are many good reasons for providing incentives to agriculturalists to address these problems in a dedicated manner. By itself, increased agricultural production is an unsatisfactory and unsustainable goal, if that increased production does not address ill-health and malnutrition. Advocacy can focus attention on specific health and nutrition benefits to which agriculture can contribute, forcing the sector to consider in greater detail who truly benefits from increased agricultural productivity and how it should change its priorities and activities accordingly.

References

Benson, T. D. 2007. "Cross-Sectoral Coordination Failure: How Significant a Constraint in National Efforts to Tackle Malnutrition in Africa?" *Food and Nutrition Bulletin* 28 (2): S323–S330.

———. 2008. *Improving Nutrition as a Development Priority: Addressing Undernutrition within National Policy Processes in Sub-Saharan Africa*. IFPRI Research Report 156. Washington, DC: International Food Policy Research Institute.

Grindle, M. S., and J. W. Thomas. 1989. "Policy Makers, Policy Choices, and Policy Outcomes: The Political Economy of Reform in Developing Countries." *Policy Sciences* 22: 213–248.

Chapter 18

Accelerating National Policymaking across Sectors to Enhance Nutrition

Robert K. N. Mwadime

Introduction

National development plans in Africa are increasingly recognizing nutrition as both essential for development and a social right. So far, however, this has not resulted in the large-scale provision of nutrition services necessary to reduce the high levels of malnutrition on the continent. Nutrition now has to feature more prominently in policymaking processes, and the resultant policies have to be translated into effective programs to achieve a significant reduction in the burden that malnutrition imposes on so many African households, communities, and nations. The experience of East Africa has relevance for policy and program design in other regions affected by malnutrition.

Sector-specific nutrition policies are fairly common. For example, policies exist for micronutrients (such as iodine), breastfeeding, infant and young child feeding, and food safety, along with supporting strategies and guidelines for implementation. Most of these policies do not require new legislation or new institutional structures.

Nutrition is not a sector. It is a cross-cutting development problem that needs to be integrated into the activities and policies of the agriculture, health, education, and sanitation and water sectors (among others), and featured in the priorities of broader agencies such as ministries of finance and gender. A need exists for coordinated nutrition-related policies that will require governments to put in place new institutional frameworks, dedicated budgets, tax breaks (or other incentives) for private-sector investment, and in some cases substantial changes in operational responsibilities and processes. These and similar initiatives will require a multisectoral commitment; they need to navigate a more complex policymaking pathway—with scrutiny from a broader set of actors—than do sector-specific policies.

This chapter is based on the author's 2020 Conference Brief, *Accelerating National Policymaking across Sectors to Enhance Nutrition* (Washington, DC: International Food Policy Research Institute, 2011).

Framework for Policymaking: Awareness, Commitment, and Resources

In relation to nutrition policy change in eastern Africa—and, more broadly, throughout the developing world—three factors are frequently noted as affecting progress: (1) awareness by senior decision leaders of the importance of nutrition to the development agenda, (2) political commitment, and (3) availability of financial resources to implement programs. All three factors must interact to produce substantive policy change effective in reducing malnutrition.

Awareness

Nutrition is rarely a top agenda item for policymakers in the region. Policy documents are drafted but not finalized, and decisions are delayed. There are three main reasons for this lack of attention.

1. Most political leaders do not recognize malnutrition when they see it. Stunting and micronutrient deficiencies are accepted as the norm rather than as problems needing urgent action, or they may be hidden from view. The adverse implications of malnutrition on child and maternal survival, intellectual development, and physical and mental productivity are not appreciated. Other issues are considered more pressing, so public nutrition policies—which policymakers would rarely object to—are dismissed as less urgent and do not get formulated or implemented.

2. Policymakers have conflicting ideas about how nutrition problems should be solved. Policy discussions are dominated by political, personal, sectoral, or other institutional interests. Negotiating the policy process takes time, and nutrition policy decisions get delayed.

3. To reduce conflict between competing interests, policymakers may be unwilling to address the underlying causes of malnutrition or to target action in the most efficient manner. Instead, second- or third-best solutions are adopted; these policies fail to reduce the number of malnourished people.

Other reasons for policymakers' possible reluctance to take public action are shown in Box 1.

Nevertheless, progress can be achieved through win–win solutions. Activities designed to serve nutritional objectives may also address other policy interests that are either political or sectoral. In the free milk program in Kenya, for example, the agriculture and education communities both saw an opportunity to promote their specific interests: dairy development and increased school enrollment.

Box 1   **Reasons for w eak Commitment to t aking Public a ction a gainst Malnutrition**

- Malnutrition is usually invisible to malnourished families and communities.

- Families and governments do not recognize the human and economic costs of malnutrition.

- Political leaders may not be aware of the rapid and cost-effective interventions available for combating malnutrition.

- There are multiple organizational stakeholders in nutrition with differing interests.

- There is not always a consensus about how to intervene to reduce malnutrition.

- Adequate nutrition is seldom treated as a human right.

- The malnourished have little voice.

- Some politicians and managers are not interested in whether nutrition programs are implemented well.

Commitment

The commitment of political leaders can be best focused on the following four endeavors.

1. *Delivering statements.* In this way, senior leaders can plant the "seed" to develop a broader political commitment to reducing malnutrition.

2. *Establishing high-level national coordination bodies to address malnutrition.* This builds political commitment and keeps the topic high on the development agenda, particularly if there are adequate human resources and budget.

3. *Improving n utrition's st atus o n t he o rganizational c hart.* This involves building respect for nutrition's importance by dedicating an adequate number of staff and slice of the budget to nutrition. Currently, in ministries of health (or other responsible agencies), nutrition is typically given a low place in the

organization, with no earmarked budget and few staff positions; nutrition objectives, especially those that require coordinated action with other sectors, are consequently neglected.

4. *Making informed appointments.* This ensures nutrition will have well-informed advocates who can effectively promote the nutrition agenda. If those appointed to lead nutrition efforts lack the necessary academic background, experience, and leadership skills, their efforts will become sidelined in the competition between sectors and subsectors to influence resource allocations.

Resources

Resource allocations are a good measure of political commitment. In fact, governments in eastern Africa tend to leave nutrition financing almost entirely to donors. In the absence of new government revenue streams, moreover, public investments are unlikely to be made for new programs to address malnutrition because decisionmakers would rather access new funding sources than reallocate their existing funds.

Policymaking and Implementation

Enacting policies requires effective implementation. Unfortunately, however, written policy and actual practice are not often congruent, due to such factors as the following:

- Implementers may resist the priorities established in a policy document, based on their own assessment of the solutions needed. Ideally, the consensus-building process necessary to formulate nutrition policy should continue through implementation.

- Policies fail to define clearly the various elements that facilitate implementation: operational structures, guidelines and standards, financial resources, human capacity, and effective follow-up and coordination.

- Countries with loose interagency coordination mechanisms (such as Kenya, Mozambique, Namibia, and Uganda) have greater difficulty planning, coordinating, and funding nutrition-related mandates.

Countries where malnutrition has been recognized more broadly as a *development problem* rather than a *health problem*—including Lesotho, Malawi, Rwanda,

FIgu RE 1 openings for effective implementation of nutrition policies in policy processes

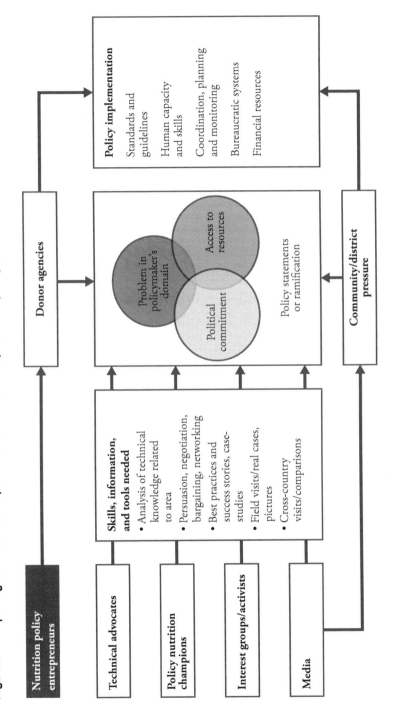

Source: Author.

and Zimbabwe—have moved toward a multisectoral response to malnutrition that involves most government ministries, the private sector, and nongovernmental organizations. To sustain this multisectoral response, some countries have established interministerial coordinating agencies for nutrition to promote the mobilization of resources, coordinate multisectoral planning, and undertake monitoring and research.

The direct and indirect activities required for effective implementation of nutrition policies are diagrammed in Figure 1, which demonstrates that *continuous advocacy, bottom-up pressure,* and *donor engagement* are all important components in achieving implementation of national programs.

Through *continuous advocacy,* policymakers are enlightened on the magnitude of malnutrition problems, their consequences, and the benefits of urgently addressing them. Unfortunately, there is often a disconnect: policymakers may not respect the advocates, who (as technical people) are their juniors in the administrative and political hierarchy. Policy champions, partnerships, and the media can cut across such barriers.

Advocacy requires multiple approaches, applied consistently and repeatedly, to communicate how the interests of different groups will be met by the nutrition policy, and it must demonstrate the real impact of action to address malnutrition. Success stories, as well as field visits to demonstrate the real suffering from malnutrition, can be very powerful tools to prompt immediate action. Improved nutrition is a fundamental element of human well-being and should be a central objective of social and economic development.

Bottom-up or grassroots pressure has been generally missing from the nutrition policymaking process. Unlike food insecurity and hunger, malnutrition is not generally identified as a priority problem by African households; communities have little understanding of the significant burden that malnutrition imposes on their well-being. Consequently, malnutrition does not create a liability for politicians. Community and civil society organizations need to mobilize people to demand services and conditions to improve their nutrition and that of their children. The grassroots communities represent a generally untapped political force that can transform the government's approach to addressing malnourishment in the region.

Donor engagement and funding have generally dictated the commitment and motivation of eastern African governments to nutrition activities. However, this means that there is no assurance of long-term local support for nutrition action. Policy implementation that depends on donor resources may instead be shut down once donor resources are exhausted, putting at great risk existing nutrition actions in eastern Africa.

TABl E 1 Nutritional problems with possible solutions and options for government action

Nutrition problem	Possible solutions	o ptions for government action
Increasing (or slow reduction in) stunting or underweight among children	Promote exclusive breastfeeding; control marketing of breast milk substitutes	Legislation on marketing of breast milk substitutes
	Improve quality of complementary foods given to young children	Local ordinances that every home must have a toilet
	Improve sanitation	Universal primary education; vocational training
	Keep girls in school	School feeding programs in areas with high dropout rates
	Increase child spacing and reduce teenage pregnancies	Age-of-marriage regulations
	Improve nutrition awareness	Access to contraceptives for teenagers
		Compulsory sex education in schools
		Incentives for FM radio stations to provide dedicated airtime for health and nutrition education
Increasing (or slow reduction in) micronutrient deficiencies	Fortify foods with micronutrients	Tax exception on fortificants used by food manufacturers (millers, vegetable oil producers, etc.)
	Diversify diets	
	Increase intake of micronutrient-dense foods	Mandatory policy to fortify all milled grain (or vegetable oil or salt) sold in the country
		Social marketing of good nutrition behaviors
Increasing overweight and obesity among school children	Increase physical education/ activity in schools	Physical education compulsory (and graded) in schools
	Improve awareness	School nutrition policy in ever school
		Food labels in local language
		Social marketing of good behaviors

Source: Author.

Recommendations

Unfortunately, there is no simple checklist for bringing a nutrition agenda to the forefront of policy concerns. The following four broad considerations should be kept in mind by policy advocates at all levels.

Box 2 w   indows of o pportunity for Nutrition Policy Change

When the leadership of the Ministry of Health changed in Kenya, the director of the National AIDS Support and Control Program immediately approached the new leaders to renew a policy request that had been languishing for months—the requirement to have a nutritionist on staff in accredited HIV/AIDS comprehensive care centers. Within days, the permanent secretary issued a memo to this effect and called for a nutritional review of the national HIV/AIDS policy. Resources were mobilized, and an additional 50 nutritionists were hired.

Recurrent droughts in Malawi mobilized the political system to invest in household food and nutrition security. The new president had promised to aggressively address the issues of malnutrition and food insecurity. Upon his election, nutrition advocates proposed a coordinating mechanism for nutrition, under the Office of the President and Cabinet. A nutrition coordinating office was established and now coordinates and monitors nutrition activities in all sectors.

---

1. *Clearly and simply define the nutrition problem, then present policy solutions.*
   a. Focus on the *problems*—for example, persistent high levels of stunting, seasonal high acute malnutrition, increasing micronutrient deficiencies, and increasing obesity. The most powerful arguments are images or descriptions of real cases showing the actual burden that malnutrition imposes on individuals and their households.

   b. Suggest several solution options for the problem. Nutrition problems are usually context specific, and solutions need to be identified based on their root causes (see Table 1). Many solutions only require new operational guidelines and standards, rather than full policy reforms.

   c. Think more broadly. In addition to food fortification, micronutrient supplementation, breastfeeding, and other direct approaches, we should frame indirect solutions that can provide the basis for sustainable reductions in childhood and maternal malnutrition. Such indirect solutions include increasing educational attainment for girls, preventing teenage pregnancy and increasing the spacing between births, improving general sanitation and hygiene, addressing gender issues (women's workload, control of household resources), changing adverse dietary and health-seeking behaviors, and improving household incomes and general welfare.

d. Be clear about the costs as well as the benefits of implementing nutrition interventions at scale. Think creatively about how to implement large-scale, simple solutions at low cost.

2. *Prepare to exploit windows of opportunity.*

Opportunities for policy change appear when senior decisionmakers become aware of nutrition problems and appreciate the need for action. Various events—including a disaster or other crisis, a sensational media report, a change in government or sectoral leadership, the political mood, or a political challenge by the opposition—may trigger attention to nutrition issues (see Box 2).

Nutrition advocates need to be prepared at such opportune moments with tools to assist the policy change process. These tools may include information about nutrition problems and the social benefits of addressing them; a pre-packaged design of programs (with budgets); and well-informed policy champions and media activists who can reinforce and channel the interest of policymakers.

3. *Redefine focus of the nutrition community.*

The nutrition community should ally with key sectors and provide them with information and program support. The community must adopt more radical approaches to increasing demand for better nutrition and engaging with community and national politics—for example, by mobilizing public awareness of systems that perpetuate malnutrition (political, cultural, or market centered). Similarly, village health workers need community mobilization skills to promote grassroots demand for local nutrition services.

The nutrition community will have to work increasingly with commercial food companies as useful partners in improving food quality. Excluding them from participating in nutrition policymaking processes, as has been the case, will result in less relevant and effective policies and programs.

The nutrition community needs to help design policies that provide vulnerable groups with greater access to services and technologies that improve their nutrition. Appropriate nutrition technologies will likely reduce dietary and nutritional differences between genders, economic groups, and rural and urban residents.

4. *Understand policymaking systems—and play politics.*

Malnutrition may reflect a range of nontechnical determinants, such as disparities in access to nutrition-related resources and services, marginalization, and cultural dynamics that disempower nutritionally vulnerable groups. These are political issues that require political engagement by the nutrition community.

Accordingly, the nutrition community needs a clear understanding of the factors that make politicians feel responsible for a particular social problem, as well as of the kinds of solutions they prefer, the language they use (and respond to), and their fears and concerns. Similarly, nutrition advocates must understand the mechanics of policy processes: how policies are made, the flow of information, and the kind of issues that are considered at various stages. Advocates need to know at what points in the year the policy process is likely to speed up or slow down, and why. They also need to know the movers and shakers personally and solicit their support.

Finally, we must be aware that, whenever a major policy is enacted, some individual, political, or institutional interests will be adversely affected. Conflict is inevitable where there are competing interests in a resource-scarce context. We should not avoid conflict, however, as we promote efforts to better meet the needs of the nutritionally vulnerable and marginalized and ensure that they and their children will live healthier, happier, and longer lives.

Chapter 19

Advocacy to Reduce Malnutrition in Uganda: Some Lessons for Sub-Saharan Africa

Brenda Shenute Namugumya

There has been increasing recognition in Sub-Saharan Africa over the past decade of the significance of malnutrition as a brake on both human and economic development and a burden in the lives of many African households. Governments are taking measures to reduce the prevalence of malnutrition among their citizens, but the problem is serious: 57 million African children under five years of age suffer from chronic malnutrition, and 6 million of them are acutely malnourished (Black et al. 2008). More broadly, micronutrient deficiencies remain persistently high.

To combat this problem, a supportive environment is being created. Several global initiatives to address young child and maternal malnutrition are now engaging with national governments in Africa. During the past two years, the African Union has fostered efforts and provided leadership for countries seeking to eliminate or reduce food and nutrition insecurity.

However, there are still few effective actions at sufficient scale to address malnutrition. A 2009 report documented growing political commitment to address malnutrition in most affected countries but also observed that improving the operational capacity to address the problem at various levels remained a key challenge—as evidenced by remarkably low national budget support for nutrition action (Engesveen et al. 2009).

Drawing from the case of Uganda, this chapter develops a model showing how advocates for improved nutrition in the countries of Sub-Saharan Africa might engage with governments and communities and move from knowledge to commitment to action in order to sharply reduce the number of malnourished people.

This chapter is based on the author's 2020 Conference Brief, *Advocacy to Reduce Malnutrition in Uganda: Some Lessons for Sub-Saharan Africa* (Washington, DC: International Food Policy Research Institute, 2011).

The focus here is on the use of advocacy to foster sustainable partnerships and implement nutrition strategies in Sub-Saharan Africa.

Nutrition Institutions and Policies in Uganda

Uganda, like most countries with a high burden of malnutrition, has seen limited progress in reducing the levels of maternal and child malnutrition over the past two decades. In a 2010 report, FANTA-2 explains that the most common forms of malnutrition in Uganda were chronic malnutrition and micronutrient deficiencies—in particular, deficiencies in iron (prevalence of 73 percent among under-fives and 49 percent among women of reproductive age) and vitamin A (20 percent among under-fives). Although micronutrient deficiencies have a major impact on health, growth, and physical development, they rarely have visible symptoms; much of the malnutrition in Uganda is thus a hidden problem. Malnutrition is a key contributor to childhood mortality in Uganda, as an underlying cause of around 150 childhood deaths every day. The long-term economic impact of this level of stunting—coupled with high levels of iron-deficiency anemia, iodine-deficiency disorders, and low birth weight—is estimated at US$310 million annually due to lost productivity, representing a 4.1 percent reduction in Uganda's gross domestic product (FANTA-2 2010).

Improving nutrition outcomes forms a core component in the health sector strategies highlighted in the Uganda National Minimum Health Care Package of the Health Sector Strategic Plan II (Ministry of Health 2005). Implementation of preventative approaches such as integrated management of childhood illness, immunization, health education, and promotion emphasizes control of communicable diseases and school and environmental health. This is reinforced by the range of nutrition initiatives funded by foreign donors either independently or through the sectors of health and agriculture. However, the scale of implementation and budget allotted is inadequate for sustainably impacting national indicators. Steps have been taken to create a policy environment conducive to addressing Uganda's nutrition and food security challenges. A review of several key policy documents setting the development priorities and strategies of the Government of Uganda—including the master development framework, the National Development Plan—shows that nutrition is included as a development concern. As in many other developing countries, however, the implementation of these strategic documents tends to be poor. There are several reasons for this, both general and nutrition-specific.

1. In Uganda there is no formal mechanism to coordinate nutrition activities among the various public and private entities that should be involved. Malnutrition is

seen as everyone's problem but no one's responsibility, resulting in a failure to take collective action.

2. There is low awareness among the relevant stakeholders of the roles and responsibilities they should take in implementing nutrition policies.

3. The general low awareness of the significance of malnutrition for Uganda's development has led to poor prioritization of nutrition issues and, in turn, low investment of financial and human resources for sustainable and broad-scale nutritional improvement.

Despite these reasons, the level of political commitment to address malnutrition in Uganda has been improving over the past three years, and the change is in part attributable to aggressive advocacy campaigns.

Building consensus among stakeholders around the nutrition issues in African countries is a key step to successful resource mobilization and to implementation of strategies and programs. Uganda's steady scaling-up of efforts to address malnutrition can serve as a model for this advocacy approach.

Recent Nutrition Advocacy in Uganda

The ministries—health, agriculture, education, gender, trade and industry, finance, and local government—that can play a role in reducing malnutrition in Uganda have not made the issue a high priority. There is no national nutrition plan and only limited human and financial capacity committed to implementation. Political leaders have little interest in or understanding of the need for nutrition activities. Indeed, until quite recently, implementation of initiatives to address malnutrition in Uganda has depended on donor-driven agendas. In 2008, however, leadership for nutrition was strengthened in both the health and agricultural sectors. Both sectors began campaigns to strengthen capacity at the central level to provide leadership for efforts to address malnutrition, and both sectors committed increased financial resources for nutrition activities. Several notable activities have resulted.

1. The health sector convened a national nutrition stakeholder forum, with several objectives: (a) to provide an opportunity for information dissemination; (b) to initiate coordination between health and agriculture sector activities; and (c) to offer a mechanism for designing improved nutrition programming. Initially external development agencies and civil society organizations (some external while others are domestic but funded mostly by external donors) contributed most of the technical and financial support for the forum; currently leadership

and budget allocation is integrated in the health sector plan for institutionalization. The forum meets on a quarterly basis with more than 70 participants from public, private, and civil society, and development partner agencies. A central objective of the forum is to develop a strong nutrition policy framework across all of the relevant sectors in order to generate better and more effective programming to address malnutrition. Similar forums at the regional level have since been organized, for planning district-level nutrition and food security activities.

2. In recent strategic planning exercises of both the health and agriculture sectors, their nutrition-focused mandates were reviewed and nutrition activities were incorporated into new sector development strategies. Various stakeholders were engaged in this consultative process, equally supported by both the health and agriculture sectors and external development agencies.

3. During the drafting of the National Development Plan and at the invitation of the National Planning Authority, a multisectoral, interagency approach successfully incorporated strategies related to nutrition and food security into five sections: health, agriculture, education, gender, trade, and finance. Nutrition-related activities were included in the Plan's investment portfolio, which prioritizes activities to receive financial support from the government or its development partners.

The aim of these advocacy efforts is to expand the set of public and private sector actors involved beyond the health and agriculture sectors. This enlarged set of stakeholders is expected to address a broader range of factors that contribute to malnutrition. Table 1 suggests benchmarks that could be applied to monitor the effectiveness of these nutrition advocacy efforts.

As part of this effort, in early 2009 a nutrition advocacy technical working group was formed for Uganda. In addition to the health and agriculture sectors, the working group participants included representatives of the education, gender, and population sectors, public agencies responsible for statistics and standards, development partners, civil society organizations, the media, and academia. The working group studied all the available data on nutrition for Uganda, developing evidence to demonstrate the need for increased public investment in improved nutrition in Uganda. The working group then developed a nutrition advocacy presentation as well as four educational briefs on the impact of nutrition on agriculture, health, education, and economic development (UGAN 2010).

Though the working group was spearheaded by the health sector, it relied heavily on financial support from external development partners and civil society organizations (all reliant on external funding) for all activities undertaken. Resources

TAb Le 1   Benchmarks for monitoring nutrition advocacy

Short term	medium term		l ong term
c reate evidence base for decisionmaking	increase demand	c hange in stunting (points per year)	Better diets (calories, proteins, fats)
• More professional dialogues on addressing malnutrition at various forums • More operational research addressing how barriers to nutrition programming can be overcome • Contextual and evidence-based media coverage on nutrition issues • Formation of multisectoral working groups to draft action plans • Participatory, multisectoral, and budgeted strategic plans • Advocacy tools developed specific to nutrition—for example, the Uganda nutrition advocacy package	• Critical mass of high-level nutrition advocacy champions— politicians, country directors, cultural and religious leaders • Increase in forums on need to address malnutrition at all levels • Nutrition included in central and district annual development plans • Increase in contextual evidence-based media coverage on nutrition issues • Increase in multisectoral demand-driven professional capacity-building forums • Resource reallocation at all levels to support nutrition • Review and update institutional curriculum to include nutrition	• Institutional restructuring to integrate nutrition in other sectors at all levels • Establishment of institution for multisectoral coordination of nutrition interventions • Review and development of cross-cutting policies and guidelines with nutrition content • Community empowerment to foster demand for nutrition programs • Specific resource allocation—both human and financial— for nutrition at all levels • High-level policy champions regularly speak about nutrition • Scale up nutrition interventions to achieve national coverage	• Increased budget allocations specifically for nutrition at all levels • Accountability forums for nutrition expenditures with high-level participation • Strong national coordination, monitoring, and evaluation for nutrition resources • Strong decentralized response capacity in place to address malnutrition

Source: Author.

for supporting advocacy activities were planned under the five-year Maternal Infant and Young Child Nutrition Plan and operational strategy. However, putting this goodwill into action remains a challenge. The meager budget allotted to the sector's nutrition unit is inadequate to support the advocacy activities. Being a multisectoral group, power struggles among sectors and inadequate ownership of developed materials tainted the working group. This is partly attributable to the failure of the health sector to raise funds for the working group.

Champions for Nutrition Advocacy

Nutrition advocacy champions, with both political and technical backgrounds, are needed at all levels to create effective political demand for better nutrition. This was a primary goal in engaging the Uganda Action for Nutrition Society and the Uganda Dietetic Association. Both associations have multisectoral membership, including high-profile professional participants like the first lady of Uganda and the vice president.

More significantly, high-level individual champions have raised the profile of nutrition in various policy forums. Such champions are able to deliver advocacy messages on the impact of malnutrition on Ugandan development in an easy and innovative manner that is understood by nonprofessionals. They have been successful both in influencing nutrition-related decisionmaking and, importantly, in breaking the silence in the political arena on nutrition issues.

Media engagement forms part of the advocacy campaign. The working group conducted a gap analysis to learn why reporting on nutrition is given low priority in Uganda; it developed a partnership with the Uganda Health Communication Alliance (an association of health journalists) to facilitate reporting on nutrition stakeholder discussions and to enable journalists to visit programs implementing nutrition interventions. Media representatives have also participated in various advocacy forums on nutrition, including activities associated with World Breastfeeding Week and workshops on the links between agriculture and nutrition.

The working group also drafted a statement to obtain public commitment to nutrition from the major candidates for Uganda's 2011 presidential election. These pledges are currently being collected, and the group will ensure that local media give significant coverage to these signed pledges. A rise has been noted in the number of stories on nutrition and food security topics in the print media and on local television. By engaging actively with journalists, nutrition advocacy efforts in Uganda are reaching large audiences at a relatively low cost.

Lessons Learned

Box 1 lists some of the recent successes with advocacy for increased public investment in nutrition in Uganda. More broadly, the agenda for action for improved nutrition has been advanced in Uganda through a range of engagements and interventions, including

- recognizing opportunities for advocacy and education in the policy landscape (for example during high-level public events and the election cycle, when the policy direction changes and creates a need for new information and strategies);

---

box 1 r   ecent o pportunities for n utrition a dvocacy in u ganda

- In August 2009, a workshop sponsored by the Uganda Academy of Sciences reached agreement on the need for increased investment in nutrition, sustainable implementation of community-based nutrition initiatives, and harmonized coordination of nutrition activities, particularly involving the agricultural sector.

- The first opportunity to use new educational materials and to exploit new media relationships arose during the July 2010 African Union Summit in Kampala. At a side event on food and nutrition, presentations on the importance of nutrition for socioeconomic development in Uganda were made and official assurances were obtained to speed up the endorsement of the pending Uganda Food and Nutrition Bill.

- Finally, at the UN Summit on the Millennium Development Goals held in September 2010, the representative of the Government of Uganda committed to reduce malnutrition in the country substantially and sustainably, under the global Scaling-Up Nutrition Initiative. This provided an opportunity for multisectoral interagency collaboration to design a Uganda National Nutrition Action Plan, focusing on young children and their mothers. Following consultations with implementers, the plan will be submitted to the Government of Uganda's cabinet for official adoption.

- drafting speeches for senior government officials that incorporate nutrition messages;

- responding to requests for presentations and documentation on improving nutrition by providing materials that demonstrate its importance to Uganda's human, social, and economic development; and

- proactively engaging with Uganda's media to ensure that messages on improved nutrition reach the target audiences, including policymakers.

Identifying and exploiting opportunities requires adequate financial resources. It was a lack of resources, in fact, that hampered the working group's efforts to promote malnutrition reduction. There were notable missed opportunities related to Global Handwashing Day, World Food Day, and World AIDS Day, as well as the Uganda Health Partners' review meetings and the political parties' planning workshops prior to the countrywide election.

Nevertheless, there is a lot of goodwill to reduce malnutrition in Uganda and Sub-Saharan Africa. Governments and their development partners have designed numerous broad programs to assist Africa's development, including improving the nutritional well-being of its citizens. However, there often is little direction for converting this goodwill into action. Thus a coordinated system for scaling up proven nutrition-improvement practices in and across each country is vital. A necessary component of such a system is careful engagement with and investment in advocacy at all levels to create demand for improved nutrition and build sustainable private and public partnerships for nutrition action.

Malnutrition is a result of failures by many different sectors in a country; combating it requires professionalism as well as a passion for attaining significant sustainable results. Change is needed in order for Uganda and other countries in Sub-Saharan Africa to reduce child and maternal malnutrition to levels where stunted children are a rarity in African communities. Advocacy is an essential tool to foster sustainable partnerships across agencies and, ultimately, to improve the performance of the sectors concerned.

The achievements realized in Uganda in recent years point to four key factors for successful nutrition advocacy.

1. Strategic networking is essential to create strong linkages and foster effective, coordinated action by the relevant agencies. Funding is required for materials and activities to sustain the network and make it effective.

2. Nutrition champions are needed at all levels and multiple sectors to promote nutrition agendas and actions. These champions should be located strategically, as indicated by an analysis of the current nutrition situation, its determinants, and its impact on health and development.

3. Stakeholder consensus is vital for successful advocacy. Ensuring that partners understand and agree with the nutrition improvement agenda is an essential first step in providing an environment conducive to resource mobilization and implementation.

4. All available nutrition advocacy opportunities must be seized. Malnutrition in Sub-Saharan Africa generally affects populations that do not vote, so the political process is unlikely to generate public investments to meet their nutritional needs. Advocates need to identify and utilize opportunities provided by national

events and high-profile meetings in order to gain policymakers' support for taking action to address malnutrition.

References

Black ,R. E., L. H. Allen, Z. A. Bhutta, L. E. Caulfield, M. de Onis, and M. Ezzati. 2008. "Maternal and Child Undernutrition: Global and Regional Exposures and Health Consequences." *Lancet* 371: 243–60.

Engesveen, K., C. Nishida, C. Prudhon, and R. Shrimpton. 2009. "Assessing Countries' Commitment to Accelerate Nutrition Action Demonstrated in PRSPs, UNDAFs and through Nutrition Governance." *SCN News* 37: 10–16.

FANTA-2 (Food and Nutrition Technical Assistance II Project). 2010. *The Analysis of the Nutrition Situation in Uganda.* Washington, DC: FANTA-2.

Ministry of Health. 2005. *Health S ector S trategic P lan II, 2 005/2006–2009/2010.* Kampala: Government of Uganda.

———. 2010. *Five-Year Nutrition Action Plan Maternal Infant and Young Child Nutrition (MIYCN).* Kampala: Government of Uganda.

UGAN (Uganda Action for Nutrition). 2010. *Economy a nd Nutrition, A n A dvocacy P ackage: Malnutrition — Uganda Is Paying Too High a Price.* UGAN Brief 4. Kampala, Uganda: UGAN.

Chapter 20

Exploring the Agriculture–Nutrition Disconnect in India

Stuart Gillespie and Suneetha Kadiyala

India is home to one-third of the world's undernourished children, with rates of child undernutrition remaining stubbornly high for decades. Undernutrition is widespread among adults, too; one-third of all Indian men and women are affected. At the same time, India is the second-fastest-growing economy in the world. Its economic growth, however, has been far less "pro-poor" than growth in other Asian countries such as China, Thailand, and Vietnam, where major strides to reduce child undernutrition have been made during similar periods of economic growth. Why has such progress somehow eluded India? What lies beneath the apparent paradox of simultaneous nutritional stagnation and sustained economic growth in India?

The Indian Enigma

Globally and historically, economic growth has played a critical role in addressing undernutrition; the rate of decline in child underweight prevalence tends on average to be around half the rate of growth of per capita gross domestic product (GDP) (Haddad et al. 2003). If this rough benchmark is applied to India, which grew at 4.2 percent per year from 1990 to 2005, the underweight prevalence would have been expected to decline by 2.1 percent a year, or by about 27 percent overall during this period. But the actual decline in these 15 years was only about 10 percent, according to National Family Health Survey (NFHS) data.

There are undoubtedly many parts to this puzzle. It is now widely recognized that nutrition outcomes are determined by a complex interaction among preconditions, including individual dietary intake and health status, household food security, caring capacity and practice, access to adequate health services, and a healthy environment—all of which are reinforced by deeper social, economic, and political processes that drive and enable them.

This chapter is based on the authors' 2020 Conference Brief, *Exploring the Agriculture–Nutrition Disconnect in India* (Washington, DC: International Food Policy Research Institute, 2011).

But one part of the puzzle surely relates to the role of the agriculture sector. Although declining in its share of India's overall GDP (at 16 percent in 2007), agriculture and allied sectors employ 52 percent of the total workforce in India, and the sector continues to play a major role in the overall socioeconomic development of the country. Through agriculture policy (including price policy), agriculture technology (including irrigation and research and development), and food marketing systems (including the creation of value chains), the agriculture sector has the potential to influence poverty reduction and the conditions under which people are employed (including time-use patterns, child labor, and exposure to hazards). It also has the potential to improve the availability of and access to diverse foods and, thereby, food consumption patterns.

Agriculture research and technology development in India have dramatically increased food production and aggregate food availability—rendering large-scale famine a rarity—yet the crisis of chronic undernutrition persists. This chapter examines this phenomenon by summarizing key nutrition outcome trends and patterns in agricultural growth and development in the country; presenting a conceptual framework for pathways between agriculture and nutrition; and using an empirical literature review to highlight the evidence for these linkages in India during the past two decades.

Trends in Nutrition Outcomes

The three rounds of the National Family Health Survey (undertaken in 1992–1993, 1998–1999, and 2005–2006) show that the prevalence of *stunting* (low height for age) among children under three years old dropped 8.1 percentage points in the 13 years between the first and third round of surveys, while *underweight* (low weight for age) prevalence declined by 7.1 percentage points. The proportion of *wasting* (low weight for height) in children declined only marginally over the same period—in fact, it actually rose significantly between NFHS-2 and NFHS-3.

Among adults, both undernutrition and anemia prevalence rates increased among women between NFHS-2 and NFHS-3, and more than one-third of married women and men in India were too thin, according to the body mass index (BMI) indicator. More than half of women and about one-quarter of men suffer from anemia.

To meet the first Millennium Development Goal, India needs to achieve an average decline of about 1 percentage point per year in the prevalence of child underweight between 2000 and 2015. Although there are substantial interstate variations in nutrition outcome trends, according to NFHS data the actual national rate of decline in underweight children in the most recent survey period has been around 0.5 percentage points per year—only half of what is required.

In addition to stagnation in undernutrition rates, India is facing a rising tide of obesity and related metabolic disorders. This double burden raises important challenges with regard to fine-tuning agricultural policies to deal simultaneously with issues of deficit, excess, and dietary imbalance.

Trends in Agricultural Development

Large-scale government investments in agriculture in the 1960s sparked India's Green Revolution. These investments resulted in improved seeds (primarily wheat and rice), subsidized inputs, infrastructure developments, increased research and extension, and new marketing policies, accompanied by relatively favorable agricultural price regimes and well-coordinated government leadership. Irrigated area doubled, fertilizer use increased sixfold, and cereal production nearly doubled. National food stocks grew, large-scale famine was all but eliminated, and rural poverty fell from 64 percent in 1967 to 50 percent in 1977, and then to 34 percent by 1986.

Since the economic reforms of the 1990s, India has seen unprecedented economic growth rates, although agriculture and allied sectors have grown much more slowly than the manufacturing and service sectors. While a falling share of agriculture in the GDP is not uncommon in a rapidly growing economy, the agriculture sector shows several disturbing trends (Bhalla and Singh 2009). The average rate of growth of agricultural yield per year has been falling steadily (at 4.4 percent between 1980 and 1990, 2.8 percent between 1991 and 1998, and 0.6 percent between 1999 and 2009). Although India ranks second worldwide in farm output, per capita daily foodgrain availability in 2006 was the same as during the drought years of the 1970s. (Concomitantly, there were rising net exports and additions to government buffer stocks.) The annual growth rate of public investment in agriculture declined from 4 percent in the 1980s to 1.9 percent in the 1990s. The parallel slowing of the poverty-reduction rate, epidemic of farmer suicides (indicative of deep agrarian distress), and virtual stagnation in nutrition outcomes nationwide highlight deep-rooted systemic problems.

Pathways between Agriculture and Nutrition

The pioneering UNICEF conceptual framework for nutrition has proved extremely useful in showing the relevance of the "food, health, and care" triad of preconditions that underpin nutritional well-being. The framework's simplicity aids communication between multiple stakeholders, but it is not necessarily optimal for highlighting specific pathways and generating testable hypotheses. Figure 1 shows a framework,

Figure E 1   Mapping the agriculture–nutrition disconnect in India

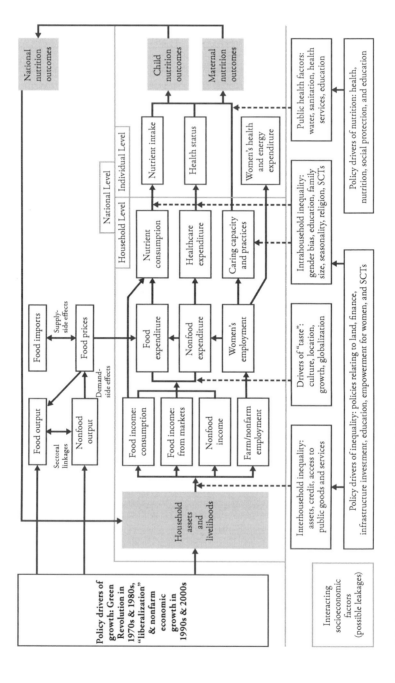

Source: Adapted by author from Headey, Chiu, and Kadiyala 2010.

developed and modified through an extensive consultative process with multiple stakeholders, that details the seven key pathways between agriculture and nutrition.

First, *agriculture as a source of food*: This is the most direct pathway by which household agricultural production translates into consumption (via crops cultivated by the household). Second, *agriculture as a source of income*: Agriculture can generate income either through wages earned by agricultural workers or through the marketed sales of food produced. For the latter, production decisions are based on tradability and the price that produce can command as a commodity, more than on its desirability for the household's own use. Third, *the link between agricultural policy and food prices*: A range of supply-and-demand factors affect the prices of various marketed food and nonfood crops, which, in turn, affect the incomes of net sellers and the ability to ensure household food security (including diet quality) of net buyers. Fourth, *income derived from agriculture and how it is actually spent*: Especially important is the degree to which nonfood expenditures are allocated to nutrition-relevant activities (for example, expenditures for health, education, and social welfare).

Pathways five through seven relate to *the increasing feminization of the labor force* and the implications this may have on (1) women's socioeconomic status, their control of resources, and their ability to influence household decisionmaking and intrahousehold allocations of food, health, and care; (2) their ability to manage the care, feeding, and health of young children; and (3) their own nutritional status, when their work-related energy expenditure exceeds their intakes, their dietary diversity is compromised, or their agricultural practices are hazardous to their health (which, in turn, may impact their nutritional status).

All these pathways are significantly modified by a range of factors, including the nature of the agricultural system and whether agricultural growth is driven largely by staples or nonstaples, by cereals or animal production. Other key modifiers include different types of inequities (gender, socioeconomic, caste, religious, rural/urban, geographical, and so forth), taste and preference, and other nutrition-relevant policies and programs.

Agriculture–Nutrition Linkages in India: What Is Known?

Despite agriculture's potential to affect nutrition in several ways, current knowledge about linkages between the two is extraordinarily weak. Studies that analyze malnutrition typically progress along three lines of inquiry: (1) consumption of calories, (2) micro- and macronutrient intakes, and (3) anthropometric measures. Studies on agriculture have tended to focus on agricultural productivity, incomes, and price trends. The paucity of unit-level data that combine information on both nutrition and agriculture is itself a form of "empirical disconnect" between agriculture and malnutrition.

Descriptive analyses relating agriculture growth to anthropometric outcomes of children and women show regional differences and variations by the nutrition indicator measured. For example, between 1992 and 2005, Andhra Pradesh, Maharashtra, Himachal Pradesh, Tamil Nadu, Kerala, Bihar, and Assam experienced fairly rapid agricultural growth and significant improvement in at least one anthropometric indicator, but improvements were uneven: Andhra Pradesh made no improvement in child stunting, Kerala made no improvement in underweight prevalence in children, and Assam and Bihar experienced a sharp increase in the prevalence of low BMI in women. Madhya Pradesh and Gujarat saw fairly strong agricultural growth and very poor anthropometric outcomes. In any such analysis, it will be important to investigate differences across entire population distributions for different indexes (stunting, wasting, underweight, and overweight) and for different people (women and children, especially).

In search of explanations for such variance, a systematic search of 15 databases was conducted. This yielded 4,545 citations, which were then screened for their relevance to the pathways described above. Only 71 of these articles—of varying scale, scope, methodology, and rigor—addressed the pathways, and most did so only partially.

The literature of the past two decades confirms the importance of engaging in agriculture as a *source of food* for producer households. But given the fluctuations in the agriculture sector (due, for example, to market volatility and seasonality), diversifying food sources seems to be important. Diversification of foods grown by a household can itself improve dietary diversity and nutrition outcomes. However, without further investments in public health and nutrition education, producing foods with high nutritional value does not necessarily lead to their increased intake by producer households, and any negative shocks tend to exacerbate the existing intrahousehold allocation bias against women.

While it is not clear if source of household income matters, income does influence food consumption patterns in India. Trends in food consumption during the past two decades show positive but declining income elasticities for calories and protein, but much higher income elasticities for fats. At the household level, the overall pattern is one of stable rice and wheat consumption for the poor, sharp declines in coarse cereal consumption, ongoing declines in pulse consumption, and rising consumption of fat. In contrast, the one nutritionally beneficial trend is the slow rise in consumption of high-value micronutrient-rich items. Persistent poverty and undernutrition among landless agricultural laborers are continuing causes of concern.

Demand for nutrients is susceptible to price changes, especially in rural areas where incomes have been stagnant. Most rural households are both producers and consumers, and the net impact of price changes on consumption is still unclear. The current evidence suggests that food prices induce changes in food-consumption patterns through both direct and cross-price effects. In the case of changes in consumption patterns of rice, wheat, coarse cereals, and pulses, which are relatively close substitutes, policies have played a critical role in driving relative price changes. For example, lack of investment in pulses and the policy bias toward wheat and rice (reflected in the large allocation of research-and-development funds, fertilizer and water subsidies, and the inclusion of rice and wheat in the country's Public Distribution System) led to the marginalization of pulse production in India.

A few studies have found that India's Public Distribution System have reduced households' vulnerability to poverty. But in light of falling calorie consumption amid excess national grain stocks, there is growing concern over inefficiency in the system. Critics argue that the problem is distributional and that the Government of India has (incorrectly) responded to the lack of purchasing power among the poor by favoring overproduction of a few staples. The literature suggests that consequent deflationary policies then hit producers as prices are pushed down and as incomes from agricultural wages fall, contributing to high undernutrition rates.

Evidence about the ways engagement in agriculture influences nutrition-augmenting actions (healthcare, sanitation, and so forth) is scant and suggests that households adjust expenditures on food, nonfood, and health items proportionally when faced with livelihood shocks and stresses.

In 2004–05, about two-thirds of the female labor force in India was employed in the agriculture sector; in rural areas, this proportion was 83 percent. India is witnessing a feminization of the agricultural workforce as men are more rapidly shifting into nonfarm sectors. Yet women's role in agriculture continues to be under-valued. Evidence to date suggests a very heavy work burden for women engaging in agricultural activities. Women are more likely to have chronic energy deficiency, which has implications for intergenerational transmission of undernutrition. The low socioeconomic status of women in India affects intrahousehold allocation of resources required for improving nutrition outcomes. It has been noted for several decades that developments in agriculture, such as its increasing commercialization, should be gender-sensitive and at the minimum not adversely affect the capacity of women to care for themselves and their children. Experiences in India and else-where show that the impact on the welfare of women and their children from an increasingly feminized agricultural labor force is determined by the extent to which women's socioeconomic status and decisionmaking power changes.

Policy and Program Implications

A detailed analysis of policy and program responses lies beyond the scope of this chapter, but some pointers are provided here, drawing on the work of the TANDI initiative (see Box 1). First, agricultural growth in India needs to be far more inclusive, if it is to benefit nutrition. Productivity in rainfed and resource-poor areas should be prioritized, and a particular focus should be applied to the farm and nonfarm rural livelihood base of small and marginal farmers. Second, diet quality and nutrition need to be recognized as key outcomes of agricultural development, with policy reforms geared to supporting credit, technology, water, and marketing for development of biofortified crops, pulses, fruits, vegetables, livestock, dairy, and fisheries. Third, and crucially, agriculture needs to become far more "gender proactive." Women's land and property rights need to be protected, and the prevailing gender bias in institutions and support systems need to be corrected. Platforms for empowering women to access agriculture-, health-, and nutrition-related resources need to be promoted, along with the provision of quality childcare facilities at work sites.

Finally, it is worth highlighting the pivotal need to identify and operationalize mechanisms and incentives for forging links among the agriculture, health, and social welfare sectors to address India's nutrition crisis. To tackle such a fundamentally multisectoral issue as undernutrition, systems of governance and convergence need to be better aligned across the sectors.

BOx 1 **tackling the agriculture–nutrition disconnect in India: the tandi Initiative**

Agricultural initiatives alone cannot solve the nutrition crisis in India but they can play a much bigger role toward that end than they have done thus far. This basic belief gave rise in January 2010 to the TANDI initiative, facilitated by the International Food Policy Research Institute (IFPRI) with funding from the Bill & Melinda Gates Foundation. The goal of TANDI is to better understand and address the failure of economic and agricultural growth to make significant inroads into reducing malnutrition in India. The initiative is promoting the establishment of a multistakeholder platform, which brings together economists, nutritionists, and other stakeholders to address key knowledge gaps and drive a change in India's nutrition policy and program processes.

Conclusion

While a substantial body of literature focusing on Indian agricultural development exists, there is an extraordinarily thin evidence base for the links between major agriculture-related institutional, technological, and policy shifts in the past two decades and the nutritional status of women and children. It is urgent that this gap be addressed so that the nature of agriculture–nutrition links or disconnects, and their variations across socioeconomic groups and regions, can be clarified. Building nationally representative panel datasets that enable this inquiry in the short and long runs is crucial. Without progress in joining empirical and information disconnects, policy gaps will remain. A commitment to evaluating the impact of agriculture on nutrition outcomes and understanding its pathways is critical if India is to realize the agriculture sector's potential to reduce undernutrition. TANDI's work to build a multistakeholder and cross-disciplinary agriculture–nutrition platform—and to identify key policy options and responses—is a major step in this direction.

references

Bhalla, G. S., and G. Singh. 2009. "Economic Liberalisation and Indian Agriculture: A Statewise Analysis." *Economic and Political Weekly* 44 (52): 34–44.

Haddad, L., H. Alderman, S. Appleton, L. Song, and Y. Yohannes. 2003. "Reducing Child Malnutrition: How Far Does Income Growth Take Us?" *World Bank Economic Review* 17 (1): 107–131.

Headey, D., A. Chiu, and S. Kadiyala. 2010. "Why Has Agricultural Development Not Contributed to Improved Nutrition in India?" Paper prepared for the conference "Ten Years of War Against Poverty," Manchester, UK, September 8–10.

Chapter 21

Bridging the Gap between the Agriculture and Health Sectors

Joachim von Braun, Marie T. Ruel, and Stuart Gillespie

As a unified set of global poverty reduction goals, the Millennium Development Goals (MDGs) in principle provide an opportunity for overcoming sectoral divides and forging effective links between agriculture and health. Both agriculture and health are important for most of the MDGs, and positive synergies could link agricultural and health policy, programming, and research in ways that would benefit both sectors and advance the MDGs as a whole. But these links have not materialized in satisfactory ways.

This chapter argues that while the MDG concept is clear on goals, it has never been clear on how to link goals to policies and on how to promote synergies between goals. A framework for linking agriculture and health in ways that alleviate poverty and hunger is missing, as is a set of policies to effectively exploit the synergies between agriculture and health. Such a framework requires an additional emphasis on context, governance, and policy tools.

Limitations of the MDGs in Fostering Action across Sectors

The MDGs have guided the planning and implementation of different development efforts. But their usefulness is limited unless they are combined with a policy framework, strategy, and implementation plan. Although they offer a shared vision of what is needed, they provide no common articulation of how to get there—and especially how to address the goals as a whole rather than through separated actions. The following limitations center on MDG1, on hunger and poverty, but they are also relevant for most other MDGs:

1. MDG discourse has been relatively silent about effective policies for achieving the goals. Economic theory emphasizes that achieving goals depends on the use

This chapter is based on material by the authors in *The African Food System and Its Interactions with Human Health and Nutrition*, edited by P. Pinstrup-Andersen (Ithaca, NY, US: Cornell University Press in cooperation with the United Nations University).

of at least as many different policy instruments as there are goals. Moreover, pursuing each goal independently may result in an inefficient portfolio of policies.

2. The monitoring process is poorly defined and lacks transparency—a situation that raises questions about the measurement of progress. It is unclear whether the process is carried out independently, and discrepancies in results raise doubts about the reliability of the estimation methods and findings.

3. Monitoring also focuses on average change, which hides important information on changes in inequality and poverty gaps. The fact that the issue of inequity is not appropriately addressed in achieving and monitoring the goals also raises an ethical issue. In Sub-Saharan Africa and Latin America, the proportion of ultra-poor—those who live on less than $0.50 a day—has increased in recent decades, and it is perfectly conceivable that progress may be made toward MDG1 while ultra-poverty and hunger continue to rise.

4. For many countries, the MDGs are unrealistic and unachievable. Cost assessments of aid needed to achieve several of the MDGs suggest that they cannot be achieved in the context of past financial assistance and likely levels of assistance in the coming years. It is also important to note that while the MDGs were formally established in 2000, progress in achieving some of the goals is measured using indicators calculated from the year 1990. Reducing poverty by one-half from 1990 to 2015 depends on growth over the full 25 years. Nearly half of that growth would need to have occurred in the decade before the signing of the Millennium Declaration; countries with little to no growth in that period are unlikely to achieve it in the 15 years from 2000 to 2015.

5. Finally, partners and countries are not accountable for meeting the needs of the poorest and hungry and for improving the delivery of public services in order to achieve MDG1. Accountability also tends to be defined by individual goals, not the whole set of MDGs. Different groups of stakeholders and development agencies tend to invest in one or two goals while largely ignoring the rest.

Bringing the Agriculture and Health Sectors Together

Intersectoral cooperation is a mechanism for generating solutions to complex problems, not an end in itself. But promoting cooperation in research and policy between two different sectors is challenging—sectoral barriers provide disincentives to collaboration, and analyses and communications across disciplines can be difficult. Cooperation requires an enabling policy environment, effective institutional arrangements, and the capacity of individuals to engage in an intersectoral dialogue. It relies on evidence generated by multidisciplinary research from credible sources.

Challenges in achieving intersectoral collaboration include

- the prevailing sectoral orientation of funding, budget control, planning, monitoring, and accountability;

- ignorance of intersectoral issues, with no one sector willing to take responsibility or advocate effectively for results;

- differences in paradigms, worldviews, mindsets, and professional language;

- competition among priorities, incentives, and decisionmaking processes;

- capacity constraints, including lack of knowledge about and training in multisectoral work, and rapid turnover of staff (technical, managerial, and political) that impedes the formation of the relationships and partnerships necessary to bridge institutional divides across sectors; and

- the tendency for students at universities and other institutions to be funneled into their respective disciplines without much exposure to peers, faculty, and professionals in other departments who share similar research interests but have a different professional language or view a common issue from a different perspective.

These challenges—and ways of confronting them—are researchable issues in themselves. Ultimately, there is a need to better understand how to promote a shared understanding that translates into integrated programs and policies for greater impact. A well-structured framework for implementing the MDGs could provide an excellent tool for integrating sectors in practice, and the effectiveness of the framework in fostering cross-sectoral collaboration and in accelerating progress in achieving the MDGs could be formally tested by research.

Despite the challenges, successful collaboration between sectors has occurred in some areas (see Box 1). It must be noted that effective intersectoral collaboration is complex and requires attention to the following lengthy list of actions and considerations:

- Facilitating early and inclusive engagement with relevant partners

- Ensuring an appropriate balance (in terms of numbers and skills) between agriculture and health stakeholders

- Recognizing the different cultures, incentives, and career structures of health and agriculture professionals

- Cultivating cross-sectoral consensus on common problems and on the mutual benefits of addressing them through joint work

- Developing innovative systems of communication between disciplines (based, for example, on agreed-upon shared values and principles, rules of engagement, and platforms for communication)

- Developing models and tools for assessing and analyzing joint problems (this work could identify appropriate indicators for monitoring and evaluation that could be linked to joint accountability for results and help highlight complete pathways from research outputs to development impacts)

- Strengthening capacity and incentives for development professionals to think and act intersectorally, whether in research, programming, policymaking, or funding of new initiatives—this might include joint training of "agri-health" professionals

- Synthesizing and promptly disseminating intersectoral research findings and experiences

How can national policy frameworks be oriented to promote synergies between agriculture and health? The following approaches—partially drawn from Bos (2006) and Bryce et al. (2008)—are promising.

- *Develop a joint metric for research and policy in agriculture and health.* Setting priorities for research and policy in agriculture and health requires a unified framework to avoid "ad hoc-ism." Two complementary approaches need to be merged: one approach that focuses on lives saved and livelihoods improved (as measured by mortality, morbidity, and disability-adjusted life years saved, for example), and another approach that focuses on economic productivity, growth, and returns to investment (as measured by human productivity and lifetime earnings, for example). In view of the different positions of health and agriculture in society and the economy, an integrated framework approach that includes both of these concepts would help generate an informed policy discourse on priority setting. Developing such a joint metric is essential for results-oriented action in both sectors.

Box 1 e xamples of Successful Agriculture and h ealth c ollaboration

Homestead food production. The linkages between agriculture and nutrition are particularly strong and direct for farmers and agricultural laborers. The work of Helen Keller International (HKI) on homestead food production in four Asian countries offers an example of agriculture's positive contributions to good nutrition. The HKI program aimed to improve the nutritional status of vulnerable members of low-income households in Bangladesh, Cambodia, Nepal, and the Philippines by promoting small-scale production and consumption of micronutrient-rich crops and small animals. As a result of the program, households are producing and consuming more micronutrient-rich foods; they are earning increased incomes from the sale of high-value products; and mothers, infants, and children have better micronutrient intakes (HKI/Asia-Pacific 2001).

Biofortification. Biofortification—the process of breeding food crops that are rich in essential micronutrients—is another agricultural strategy with proven benefits for health and nutrition. Orange-fleshed sweet potato (rich in vitamin A), for example, represents a successful agriculture and health partnership that has had well-documented impacts on vitamin A intake and status of young children in Mozambique (Low et al. 2007 and Hotz et al. 2011).

Irrigation and malaria control. Irrigation brings higher agricultural yields and incomes but can heighten the risk of malaria transmission, thus decreasing agricultural productivity. Successful partnerships between agriculture and health have allowed implementation of preventive measures to control malaria while modifying or manipulating agricultural water systems. Options include location-specific drainage techniques, intermittent wetting and drying of rice fields, alternation of rice with a dryland crop, and use of livestock as "bait" for mosquitoes (Mutero et al. 2005).

Agriculture and HIV/AIDS response. The majority of people affected by HIV and AIDS depend on agriculture, and their livelihoods are undermined by the disease in many countries. There is tremendous scope for agricultural policy to become more HIV-responsive and further both health and agricultural goals. For example, to overcome the lack of land and labor often facing AIDS-affected households, the Livelihoods Recovery through Agriculture Programme, implemented in Lesotho in 2002 by CARE and the Ministry of Agriculture, promotes production of crops with high nutritional content on small plots of land close to the home. Fifty-three percent of participants reported that they had stabilized or increased their food production (Abbot et al. 2005).

- *Create incentives for results-oriented intersectoral collaboration.* Governments can create incentives for results-oriented intersectoral collaboration that benefits the national good over and above strict sectoral division. These incentives would have to emanate from the highest policymaking level, such as the prime minister's office, and have the support of the ministry of finance (which would allocate financial resources for proposed intersectoral actions).

- *Apply incentives and build capacity at the local level.* Incentives—financial or otherwise—would need to apply at the local levels where implementation occurs. Because key decisions about priorities and resource allocation are often made at subnational levels, local as well as national capacity to develop contextually appropriate interventions will need to be strengthened.

- *Implement multisectoral policy reviews.* Multisectoral policy reviews could be undertaken to harmonize existing policies, identify opportunities for reciprocal action to address each other's concerns, and formulate new policies that support the concept of intersectoral collaboration. For example, countries with increasing water scarcity could formulate policies for water's optimal use in agriculture and simultaneously ensure that this resource is used in ways that protect the health of agricultural producers, their families, and the consumers of products cultivated with wastewater (Bos 2006). Such reviews could also identify perverse policies— that is, sectoral policies that contradict and counteract each other. An HIV lens, for instance, could be applied to agricultural policies to ensure that they do not inadvertently provide the conditions for more rapid spread of HIV infection or reduce households' options for responding to the impacts of AIDS (for example, agricultural diversification is associated with resilience and a strengthened ability to respond to AIDS) (Gillespie and Kadiyala 2005).

- *Carry out health impact assessments.* Health impact assessments should be undertaken (along with environmental impact assessments) to ensure that the health impacts of any new agricultural development project or new agricultural policy are considered in a timely fashion and that a public health management plan incorporates intersectoral action. This approach also requires bilateral and multilateral development agencies to review their decisionmaking criteria for projects ahead of time and adopt policies that ensure that health safeguards are incorporated.

Conclusion

The current approach toward achieving the MDGs needs an overhaul, and planning beyond the MDGs offers opportunities for more comprehensive approaches to improving human well-being. To realize this potential, it is important to stop singling out individual MDGs and instead to start recognizing the linkages among them and their functional relationships and interdependence. Strategic use and strengthening of the linkages between agriculture and health offer particularly strong opportunities for achieving poverty reduction and health goals in many low-income countries. Exploiting these opportunities requires a new initiative for evidence-based and knowledge-intensive action across the agriculture and health sectors.

References

Abbot, J., M. Lenka, P. J. Lerotholi, M. Mahao, and S. Mokhamaleli. 2005. "From Condoms to Cabbages: Rethinking Agricultural Interventions to Mitigate the Impacts of HIV/AIDS in Lesotho." Paper presented at the International Conference on HIV/AIDS and Food and Nutrition Security: From Evidence to Action, Durban, South Africa, April.

Bos, R. 2006. "Opportunities for Improving the Synergies between Agriculture and Health." In *Understanding the Links between Agriculture and Health*, edited by C. Hawkes and M. T. Ruel, 2020 Vision Focus 13, no. 16. Washington, DC: International Food Policy Research Institute.

Bryce, D. Coitinho, I. Darnton-Hill, D. Pelletier, and P. Pinstrup-Andersen. 2008. "Maternal and Child Undernutrition: Effective Action at National Level." *Lancet* 371 (9611): 510–26.

Gillespie, S. R., and S. Kadiyala. 2005. *HIV/AIDS and Food and Nutrition Security: From Evidence to Action.* Food Policy Review 7. Washington, DC: International Food Policy Research Institute.

HKI (Helen Keller International)/Asia-Pacific. 2001. *Homestead Food Production: A Strategy to Combat Malnutrition and Poverty.* Jakarta, Indonesia.

Hotz, C., C. Loechl, A. de Brauw, P. Eozenou, D. Gilligan, M. Moursi, B. Munhaua, P. van Jaarsveld, A. Carriquiry, and J. V. Meenaksi. 2011. "A Large-Scale Intervention to Introduce Orange Sweet Potato in Rural Mozambique Reduces the Prevalence of Inadequate Vitamin A Intakes among Children and Women." *British Journal of Nutrition.* Accessed February 7, 2012. FirstView online edition: http://dx.doi.org/doi:10.1017/S0007114511005174.

Low, J., M. Arimond, N. Osman, B. Cunguara, F. Zano, and D. Tschirley. 2007. "A Food-Based Approach Introducing Orange-Fleshed Sweet Potatoes Increased Vitamin A Intake and Serum Retinol Concentrations in Young Children in Rural Mozambique." *Journal of Nutrition* 137 (5): 1320–1327.

Mutero, C. M., F. Amerasinghe, E. Boelee, F. Konradsen, W. van derHoek, T. Nevondo, and F. Rijsberman. 2005. "Systemwide Initiative on Malaria and Agriculture: An Innovative Framework for Research and Capacity Building." *EcoHealth* 2 (1): 11–16.

Chapter 22

Governing the Dietary Transition: Linking Agriculture, Nutrition, and Health

Robert Paarlberg

The best approach to finding positive synergies among agriculture, nutrition, and health may depend on a country's position in the dietary transition—from a diet low in both calories and micronutrients (Stage One) to a diet that provides adequate basic energy for most people but an inadequate balance of nutrients (Stage Two) to an affluent diet that begins to provide excessive calorie energy, which can lead to health problems linked to obesity (Stage Three). As societies move through this dietary transition, government's relative importance and most essential functions will change. A common theme at all three stages is women's essential role within households, often as food producers and almost always as the primary caregivers to small children.

In Stage One countries, the best way to capture positive synergies across sectors will be to provide missing public goods, especially rural public goods. Agricultural societies cannot advance without roads, power, transport, and rule of law—as well as schools and clinics—in the countryside. In the absence of these public goods, private investors will not come into the area, and citizens—especially smallholder farmers in the countryside—will remain caught in a poverty trap. The payoff from public goods investments at Stage One can be seen across various sectors. For example, rural roads that reduce transport costs simultaneously deliver both productivity gains for farmers (by lowering the cost of purchased inputs and reducing marketing costs) and health gains for young children (by improving access to clinics).

Cross-sector links should be considered when making these public investments (for example, when determining sites for new roads, power lines, irrigation systems, or health clinics), but most of the actual synergies between the sectors will not be "administered" by governments; instead they will be captured privately when local

This chapter is based on the author's 2020 Conference Paper, *Governing the Dietary Transition: Linking Agriculture, Nutrition, and Health* (Washington, DC: International Food Policy Research Institute, 2011).

communities, nongovernmental organizations (NGOs), private firms, and individual households make use of the new public goods. These actors are typically better informed than governments regarding individual or local cross-sector impacts.

In Stage Two countries, the task shifts from public goods provision to targeted service delivery. A large share of the essential public goods will already be in place, private investment will have begun to come in, and most citizens will have escaped the poverty trap. Significant economic growth will be under way, and at this stage the challenge of good governance across sectors switches to assisting those not yet benefitting from the growth process. A number of cross-sector services will be needed by these citizens, including agricultural extension, child and maternal health services, nutritional supplementation, food fortification, nutrition education, and perhaps food-based income transfers. Public delivery of these services requires a substantial and sustainable mobilization of budget resources, capable institutions, skilled administrators, and an abundance of reliable data, but most Stage Two countries will be rapidly gaining these things. Interministerial information sharing will be necessary but not sufficient for success. Cross-sector communication within government must be supplemented by an appropriate division of labor between central and local government, government and industry, and government and community-based organizations and NGOs. The challenge is to deliver essential agricultural, health, and nutrition services to those at risk of being left behind without interrupting a continued expansion of private investment and private service delivery.

In Stage Three countries, where economic well-being is usually widespread, the preponderance of both investment and service needs will be provided almost entirely by the private sector. At this stage, the challenge of good governance becomes one of regulating this larger and more influential private sector. For example, modern commercial farming practices that carry occupational or public safety risks, including off-farm or downstream environmental hazards, will require careful regulation in the public interest. Food manufacturers, wholesalers, retailers, and restaurants will need public regulation as well.

Stage One: Delivering Public Goods to Fight Chronic Undernutrition

Stage One countries struggling with chronic undernutrition linked to poverty must give first priority to public investment needs. In these countries, especially in rural areas, critical public goods are frequently undersupplied, making it impossible for households, local communities, and private firms to play an effective role either within or across the three sectors of concern. Smallholder farmers or herdsmen will typically make up a majority of rural dwellers, and, without increased access to markets, improved technologies, health services, and schooling, the productivity of their labor will remain low. If labor productivity is low, income will also be low, thereby placing nutrition and health at risk. Public investment will be an essential first step out of this poverty trap.

In these Stage One countries (including most countries in Sub-Saharan Africa), essential rural public goods are often poorly supplied, including farm-to-market roads, water, electrical power, clinics, and schools. Rural road systems in Africa are primitive, with 70 percent of all rural citizens living more than a 30-minute walk away from the nearest all-season road (Sebastian 2007). In these rural areas, there is virtually no electrical power, health clinics are sparse and poorly equipped, and education is rudimentary. A majority of adult farmers in Africa, who tend to be women, cannot read or write in any language. In Nigeria, one of Africa's richest countries, only 31 percent of rural citizens have access to an improved water source, 35 percent to electricity, 41 percent to an all-season road within 2 kilometers of their homes, and 53 percent to improved sanitation. In Ethiopia, only 11 percent of rural dwellers live within one mile of an all-season road, only 11 percent have access to improved water, and only 2 percent have access to electricity (World Bank 2008). In these underserved rural settings, good governance requires much more than government official's being able to communicate with each other across sectors. The job of the state in the countryside is not so much to "see all aspects of the picture" as it is to change the picture entirely by providing impoverished communities with roads, power, schools, clinics, and rule of law.

Stage One countries are often tempted to skip over the investment problem and move immediately into public service delivery or regulation. Moving too quickly or too deeply into these other areas can overwhelm the limited fiscal and administrative capacities of Stage One countries. This was a lesson learned in the 1960s and 1970s when some donors promoted ambitious multisector health and nutrition planning efforts in poor countries. During the 1970s, the United States Agency for International Development funded the creation of some 26 nutrition planning entities in the developing world. These efforts faltered when the nutrition units remained understaffed, underfunded, and capable of little more than some data generation and analysis. Most governments at that time could not recruit a sufficient number of trained nutritionists to ensure adequate representation for this specialty in each relevant ministry, and the planning models often required data and test results that did not exist. In the end, the established ministries pursued their own agendas as before while the nutrition institutes remained isolated and powerless (Field 1987).

In Stage One countries, the best way to capture positive synergies across sectors may not be from the top down, but through nongovernmental institutions. The breeding of orange-fleshed sweet potatoes (OFSP) to address vitamin A deficiencies, for example, was led by the International Potato Center (CIP). Thereafter, a nutrition-focused NGO, Helen Keller International (HKI), introduced OFSP widely to local communities. In one province in Mali, more than 80 percent of adult women consumed OFSP at least once a week during the harvest period (HKI 2011).

Stage Two: Shifting to Targeted Public Service Delivery

For countries at Stage Two in the dietary transition, basic public goods (such as roads, power, water, and public health infrastructure) are in place or coming into place in most regions, thereby drawing in private investment and stimulating economic growth. For most citizens in these countries, adequate staple food supplies are affordable, and the biggest nutrition challenge is increasing micronutrient intake through dietary diversification. Improved farm performance and a rising middle class provide opportunities and incentives for private companies (such as food industries and supermarkets) to supply healthier and more nutritious products. The capacity of the state has also grown—thanks to the greater wealth of the society—which can boost tax revenues; human capital has improved thanks to urbanization and increased investments in tertiary education. Meanwhile, as the share of the population employed in farming declines in these countries, automatic spillover gains from farm productivity into improved nutrition and health will eventually decline as well.

At this intermediate stage, the central problem of cross-sector governance shifts from simple public investment to targeted public service delivery. Some categories of citizens are not able to participate in the income, nutrition, and health gains made possible by the growing private sector (for example, the ultra-poor or people in communities marginalized by language, race, or ethnicity). For these citizens, the state must provide a supplemental channel of service delivery. Smallholders in the farming sector require extension services and technical assistance to diversify their production into the higher-value crops now demanded by the growing urban sector. The urban poor require a food-security safety net in the form of cash or in-kind transfers, perhaps conditioned by cross-sector activities such as school or clinic attendance for children. Other services the state can deliver include supplementation, industrial food fortification, or education on breastfeeding. Governments at this stage are more likely to have both the fiscal and the administrative means to deliver such services with appropriate targeting.

Administrative capacity and effectiveness increase at Stage Two, but so do the barriers to interagency coordination as administrative functions become more specialized. Specialized training often breeds disconnection and jurisdictional competition between ministries. When the Government of China developed its first National Fortification Alliance (NFA) to qualify for funding from the Global Alliance for Improved Nutrition (GAIN) program, it excluded representatives from its ministry of agriculture (Juma et al. 2007). In Sri Lanka, at one point, nutrition-ists in the Ministry of Health refused to work with the Food and Nutrition Policy Planning Division (FNPPD) in the Ministry of Plan Implementation because that unit was headed by an agriculturalist rather than a nutritionist or medical doctor (Levinson 2002). Parallel disconnections driven by specialization are also manifest at the international level between, for example, the Food and Agriculture Organization of the United Nations (FAO), the World Health Organization (WHO), and UNICEF. With sufficient political leadership, however, effective cross-sector work can nonetheless proceed at Stage Two. Thailand's National Nutrition Programme, for example, includes multiple subprograms to address healthy eating habits among children and adults, including both monitoring and control of deficiencies of nutrients such as iodine, food fortification and supple-mentation, nutrition labeling, nutrition education, immunization, environmental sanitation and deworming, and a community-based integrated approach to food security. As Thailand now moves toward Stage Three of the dietary transition, these efforts are also moving toward the prevention of degenerative chronic diseases linked to overnutrition by promoting increased fruit and vegetable consumption, moderating salt intake, and monitoring the amount and quality of fat used. One key to Thailand's success has been high-level political commitment from the king, queen, and prime minister (WHO 2007).

Political leadership from the top was also critical to Brazil's widely credited multisector Zero Hunger strategy (*Fome Zero*), launched in January 2003. This initiative has now grown to include 30 programs and activities involving more than 10 ministries plus participation by state and municipal governments and the civil society. As of 2006, according to FAO, Brazil had used this program to reduce the nation's undernourished population from 17 million to 11.9 million (FAO 2009). Rather than trying to institutionalize cross-sector perspectives within existing ministries, the *Fome Zero* initiative was designed and launched by the Office of the President outside of traditional administrative channels.

In some Stage Two countries at the local level, NGOs and international NGOs are often best positioned to fill capacity deficits and help capture synergies across sectors. For example, in Bangladesh, Helen Keller International has been promoting homestead food production by providing seeds and seedlings for fruit and vegetable gardens as well as nutrition education; as of 2003, these efforts had reached more than 4.7 million individuals in Bangladesh. In this program, a strong synergy between food production and nutrition is captured directly because children in families with developed gardens consume 60 percent more vegetables than those in households without gardens (Iannotti, Cunningham, and Ruel 2009). Targeting this program toward women has been especially successful. Homestead vegetables grown by women have a higher payoff for nutrition and health because they are more likely to be fed directly to children in the household and any income they bring in is more likely be invested in the health of children.

NGOs in Bangladesh have also found many ways to partner with the government when delivering cross-sector services to targeted populations. BRAC, a rural development organization, uses resources provided by the Bangladesh Bank to provide low-interest loans to tenant farmers who are often excluded from credit markets for lack of collateral security. BRAC also uses its village organization systems to deliver agricultural extension services to the rural poor (for example, by encouraging dietary diversification through vegetable production) and also partners with the Bangladesh Rice Research Institute and the Bangladesh Agricultural Research Institute to conduct applied agricultural research.

Stage Three: Private-Sector Expansion and a Growing Need for Regulation

During Stage Three in the dietary transition, the leading challenge of good governance shifts from public investment and public service delivery to public regulation. This is due to the much larger role now being played by private investors and large corporations—such as food, agribusiness, and pharmaceutical companies—as product manufacturers and service providers. At this third stage in the dietary transition, the agricultural sector will be highly productive, highly diverse, and sufficiently capitalized to secure most of the investment, lending, and research support it needs from private sources. Public research and extension systems will remain active, but with a role steadily shrinking relative to private companies in the seed, chemical, and machinery sectors. In the nutrition and health sectors, the higher affluence of most citizens will likewise be enough to stimulate private investments to deliver a much wider variety of healthy foods and medical services. The abundance of affordable food in these societies relative to income, however, when accompanied by transitions away from physical labor and structured eating, will eventually trigger a new diet-related threat to health: a growing prevalence of obesity.

In Stage Three countries, the most important cross-sector governmental task shifts from service delivery to regulation, especially public health and safety regulation of farm practices, food companies, food retailers, restaurants, pharmaceutical companies, hospitals, and medical insurers; environmental safety also needs be monitored. As always, it will help if regulatory policy actions in one sector take into account positive or negative synergies with other sectors. Yet the major risk at Stage Three is not an inattention to cross-sector linkages but rather the political "capture" of regulators by the private industries being regulated (Stigler 1971).

We can illustrate this danger by considering the weak regulatory response of the US government to date to the country's worsening obesity crisis, due to private industry resistance. One clear source of this crisis has been excessive calorie intake from beverages, including juices, dairy drinks, alcohol, and especially sweetened soft drinks. Beverages provide Americans twice as many calories today as they did in 1965, with more than two-thirds of the increase coming from sweetened fruit juices and soft drinks.

There is no federal taxation of sweetened beverages in the United States, even though public health advocates have long called for such taxes to both discourage soft drink consumption and help pay the public cost of managing its consequences. The American Beverage Association—the organization that represents the beverage industry—spent US$18.9 million on lobbying in 2009 to stop a proposed small tax on the sale of sweetened soft drinks that would have helped pay for the US federal health bill.

The beverage industry in the United States has also gained excessive influence inside the executive branch of the federal government. The Food and Drug Administration (FDA) has declined to require that the amount of sugars or calories per container (not per serving) be included on cans and bottles. Regulatory capture by food and beverage industry groups is also visible within the United States Department of Agriculture (USDA). Even though it performs valuable nutrition functions, the USDA also houses a nonprofit corporation called Dairy Management Inc, which is dedicated to increasing the consumption of dairy products, including cheese. Americans already eat an average of 33 pounds of cheese a year—nearly triple the level consumed in 1970; it has become the largest source of saturated fat in American diets.

Taking an integrated or multisector approach to governance is not always an adequate solution at Stage Three. For example, every five years the US Congress enacts a cross-sector policy measure, known as the farm bill, that contains both a farm and a nutrition policy component, but the impact for each sector falls well short of good governance. The farm programs include poorly targeted income subsidies to wealthy commercial growers that waste taxpayer money and distort markets. President George W. Bush actually tried to veto the 2008 farm bill on the grounds that it was wasteful, but Congress still enacted it by wide majorities in both houses. The nutrition programs it enabled provide a valuable consumption subsidy to low-income citizens, but some of the programs are not necessarily well tailored to improve nutrition. The largest federal nutrition program, the Supplemental Nutrition Assistance Program (SNAP), enables 40 million participants to use the benefits they receive to purchase candy, soft drinks, and junk food. When proposals are made to eliminate sugary soft drinks from eligibility for purchase under this program, the beverage industry mobilizes to turn those proposals aside (Hartocollis 2010).

Recommendations

Does good governance have any one common feature for all three stages of the dietary transition? What matters most at each stage for capturing positive synergies is not administrative capacity, information sharing, or even strong leadership. Consistently, the key to success is an often overlooked element: the empowerment of parents—especially mothers—to provide better care for their children. When it comes to health and nutrition, those most exposed to risk are usually young children, and the agent best positioned to manage this risk is almost always the child's mother. What governance resources do mothers need to perform their parental tasks at various stages in the dietary transition? Arguably the most important resource will be education for girls and women. We have known for decades that women with more education exhibit behaviors that are more child-centered and lead to better feeding practices, better-nourished children, and healthier children. This is true at Stage One for young women in poor rural communities, at Stage Two for women beginning to seek employment outside of the home, and at Stage Three for those disadvantaged by minority status. Good governance across the agriculture, nutrition, and health sectors, then, must begin with meeting the educational needs of young women.

References

FAO (Food and Agriculture Organization of the United Nations). 2009. *A Reference for Designing Food and Nutrition Security Policies: The Brazilian Fome Zero Strategy.* Santiago, Chile: FAO Regional Office for Latin America and the Caribbean.

Field, J. O. 1987. "Multisectoral Nutrition Planning: A Post-Mortem." *Food Policy* (12): 15–28.

Hartocollis, A. 2010. "Unlikely Allies in Food Stamp Debate." *New York Times,* October 16.

HKI (Helen Keller International). 2011. "Biofortification: Orange-Fleshed Sweetpotatoes." www.hki.org/reducing-malnutrition/biofortification/orange-fleshed-sweetpotatoes.

Iannotti, L., K. Cunningham, and M. Ruel. 2009. *Improving Diet Quality and Micronutrient Nutrition: Homestead Food Production in Bangladesh.* IFPRI Discussion Paper 928. Washington, DC: International Food Policy Research Institute.

Juma, C., R. Paarlberg, C. Pray, and L. Unnevehr. 2007. "Patterns of Political Support and Pathways to Final Impact." *AgBioForum* 10 (3): 201–207.

Levinson, J. 2002. "Searching for Home: The Institutionalization Issue in International Nutrition." Background Paper. World Bank-UNICEF Nutrition Assessment. Washington, DC, and New York: World Bank and UNICEF.

Sebastian, K. 2007. "GIS/Spatial Analysis Contribution to 2008 WDR: Technical Notes on Data and Methodologies." Background paper for the *World Development Report 2008*. Washington, DC: World Bank.

Stigler, G. 1971. "The Theory of Economic Regulation." *Bell Journal of Economics and Management Science* 3: 3–18.

WHO (World Health Organization). 2007. "Food and Nutrition Policy and Plans of Action." Report prepared for the WHO-FAO Intercountry Workshop, Hyderabad, India, December.

World Bank. 2008. *The Little Data Book on Africa 2007*. Washington, DC.

Leveraging Agriculture for Improving Nutrition and Health: The Way Forward

Shenggen Fan, Rajul Pandya-Lorch, and Heidi Fritschel

The world confronts enormous challenges related to hunger and malnutrition. At the same time, it faces many opportunities, including agriculture's resurgence on the development agenda. The question is how to use these opportunities to leverage agriculture for improving nutrition and health. Broadly speaking, reshaping agriculture for better nutrition and health will require steps in four main areas: filling knowledge gaps, ensuring that the three sectors do not work at cross-purposes, seeking out and scaling up innovations and successes, and creating an environment for cooperation.

The Challenge

The linkages between agriculture, nutrition, and health seem obvious: adequate levels and qualities of food produced and consumed promote good nutrition and robust health. The reality, however, is that patterns of food production and consumption vary widely around the world and the positive linkages between agriculture, nutrition, and health are not realized. Despite the large role that agriculture has played in the past, a number of pressing problems in the areas of agriculture, nutrition, and health are evident. These problems include the following:

- Nearly a billion people now go hungry every day, unable to access the food they need for energy and growth. Several billion suffer from deficiencies in micronutrients like iron, vitamin A, and zinc (FAO 2010). Hunger and poor nutrition have severe and sometimes fatal consequences for people's health, especially for women and children. These consequences can include significantly greater susceptibility to a range of infectious diseases. At the same time, problems related to

This chapter is a synthesis of IFPRI's conclusions on the policy consultation process linked to the conference "Leveraging Agriculture Toward Improving Nutrition and Health" held February 10–12, 2011, in New Delhi, India. The chapter was designed to stimulate international debate on the way forward and does not imply any endorsement by the conference participants or the cosponsors.

"overnutrition" are burgeoning in many parts of the world. Obesity and chronic diseases like heart disease and diabetes are on the rise, even in settings where hunger is also common.

• Agriculture is dominated by smallholders—many of whom suffer from poverty, malnutrition, and poor health—and faces environmental challenges. In some regions, smallholder agriculture is not growing fast enough to keep up with rising demand for food and to provide farmers with adequate incomes. Intensification of agriculture is a must to feed an increased world population, yet agricultural intensification brings its own risks for people's health, including zoonotic diseases, food- and water-borne diseases, occupational hazards, and environmental damage that puts people and the planet at risk. Women, who make up the majority of workers on smallholder farms, are particularly vulnerable, because they are also responsible for food and nutrition security and care for the family.

• Stress on natural resources, especially water resources—exacerbated by climate change—may cause farmers to adopt farming practices that are harmful to their own health and to the health of consumers and that are ultimately not sustainable.

Addressing these problems will require solutions to be developed at the intersection of the agriculture, health, and nutrition sectors. Much has been learned in recent years about how the three sectors are connected—with important implications for people's well-being and overall economic development. Nonetheless, significant information and knowledge gaps remain. Many policymakers and practitioners in the agriculture, nutrition, and health sectors continue to work in isolation despite the potentially strong synergies among initiatives to improve nutrition and health through agriculture.

Faster progress must be made in the drive for adequate food, good nutrition, good health, and sustainable agricultural growth, but the three sectors must work together to minimize the negative links among them and maximize the positive synergies. The policy consultation process "Leveraging Agriculture for Improving Nutrition and Health" points the way to some first steps along this path, beginning with an effort to learn more about the links and the implications for policy and delivery on the ground.

Fill the Knowledge Gaps

• *Learn more about how different patterns of agricultural growth affect nutrition and health.* To design the most effective policies, we still need to know more about how much and what type of agricultural growth is best for nutrition and health.

For example, must agricultural growth pass a certain threshold to contribute to nutrition and health? Should investments focus on staple crops, high-value crops, or livestock? How can agricultural growth facilitate greater dietary diversity? What conditional factors—such as land distribution, education, women's status, producer and consumer market structures, and rural infrastructure—do the most to leverage agricultural growth for nutrition and health? Do the links among agriculture, nutrition, and health operate differently in countries at different stages of development? What incentives need to be put in place to ensure that increased farmer income translates into better health and nutrition? We need to capture the lessons learned from small-scale projects and encourage better monitoring and evaluation so that the evidence base is stronger and can be used by others.

- *Invest in research, evaluation, and education systems capable of integrating information from all three sectors.* Better-integrated research and evaluation tools and incentives will promote policymaking processes and learning that cross the agriculture, nutrition, and health sectors. For instance, it would be useful to mainstream the nutrition dimension in farming system research. Universities should encourage a more multidisciplinary approach to break down the barriers and help students—the practitioners and leaders of the future—and faculty build knowledge and relationships across the sectors. Donors and governments need to invest in reducing critical gaps in human and institutional capacity while stepping up investments in projects and evaluations. Financial incentives to promote multidisciplinary research should take into account policy relevance in more than one sector. To have the greatest impact on policy, research results should be communicated across sectoral boundaries.

- *Fill the gap in governance knowledge at the global, national, and community levels.* More remains to be learned about how to maximize the synergies among the three sectors using policies, investments, regulations, and other tools of governance.

Do No Harm
- *Mitigate the health risks posed by agriculture along the value chain.* Agricultural strategies should seek to control the agriculture-associated diseases and occupational hazards that are exacerbated by agricultural intensification. New agricultural developments should be subject to health impact assessment (HIA), which can identify health hazards and risks at the design and construction phases when cost-effective safeguards can be incorporated. Also needed are improved production and processing practices, such as better food safety practices and

water management, as well as cost-effective technologies that help smallholder farmers minimize the risk of health hazards. Advances in health-risk assessment and management promote incremental improvements through a multiple barrier approach. This provides a strong basis for public health officials to participate in disseminating information on health risks and solutions along the value chain.

- *Design health and nutrition interventions that contribute to the productivity of agricultural labor.* Nutrition interventions such as home-based gardens can both improve nutrition and raise agricultural production. HIV/AIDS interventions can be designed to take account of losses of household labor and minimize disruptions to household production.

- *Look carefully at the downstream effects of subsidies for production or consumption on consumers' nutrition and health.* Although policymakers often use nutrition to justify agricultural subsidies, in some cases subsidies may result in patterns of agricultural production and distribution that ultimately hurt people's nutrition and health. Across-the-board, untargeted consumer subsidies, for example, may help hungry people to acquire more food but, over time, may distort their consumption choices and crowd out public investments that would do more to boost nutrition and health.

Seek Out and Scale Up Innovative Solutions

- *Scale up successful interventions.* Some interventions that address the goals of all three sectors have already been tried both at the project level and at the country level—for example, homestead food production in Bangladesh (see Chapter 16), homegrown school feeding in Brazil, the National Nutrition Program in Thailand (see Chapter 22), and biofortification in Mozambique and Uganda (see Chapter 10). It is important to better understand the most cost-effective ways for agriculture and health to deliver improved food security and nutritional outcomes. What works in a particular context and why? These efforts offer opportunities for adapting and scaling up successes and learning from failures.

- *Design agriculture, nutrition, and health programs with cross-sectoral benefits.* Integrated programs can be designed to take advantage of synergies among the three sectors. For example, increased intercropping with nitrogen-fixing crops such as lentils could reduce agricultural inputs, restore soil fertility, and generate nutritional benefits for people. Gender-sensitive programs that consider the synergies and trade-offs between women's roles in agricultural production and childcare can promote positive nutrition and health outcomes. Food-based approaches and horticultural remedies used to treat poor nutrition can also do a great deal to improve health. Price policies can be used to promote consumption of more nutritious foods. Biofortification of staple crops can significantly improve the nutrition and health status of vulnerable groups, particularly women and children. Civil society actors such as nongovernmental organizations can bring indigenous knowledge about agriculture, nutrition, or health to bear on projects in other sectors.

- *Incorporate nutrition into value chains for food products.* The private sector plays an integral role in forming value chains and needs to have proper incentives, stemming from consumer demand, government intervention, or both, to include nutrition considerations at each stage of the chain. Improved nutrition results not only from greater volumes of food production on farms, but also from the way food commodities are handled in the postfarm segments of value chains. Processing can enhance year-round availability of products with high nutrient value. Fortification during postharvest processing can improve nutrient content or availability. Transport and storage improvements can reduce postharvest losses and deterioration of the nutritional quality of foods. Efficient post-farm handling can reduce costs and retail prices, thus increasing access for poor consumers. For underutilized crops rich in nutrients, value chains can be created to promote their conservation, cultivation, marketing, and consumption.

- *Use all available levers for change.* Science and technology levers, as well as economic, social, and governance levers, are important for maximizing agriculture's contribution to nutrition and health. Science and technology levers could include innovations along the whole value chain. Plant and livestock breeding can increase both availability of and access to food. Food-processing technologies can reduce storage losses and increase nutrient value. Reducing transport costs can make food more affordable as well as accessible, especially for poor urban populations. Economic levers could include policies related to markets, trade, prices, and investment. Social levers could include education and activities to promote behavioral change. Governance levers could include incentives and institutional arrangements, as well as inclusion of marginalized and excluded groups—especially women, who are at the nexus of the agriculture, nutrition, and health sectors. Political levers can also be used to generate leadership that galvanizes different sectors to work together effectively and to learn more about prioritizing and sequencing actions and investments to link the three sectors.

- *Increase consumers' nutrition literacy and highlight the consequences of dietary choices.* Consumer awareness campaigns, such as nutrition literacy programs in villages, can increase poor people's knowledge of and demand for nutritious food. More consumption of nutritious foods can not only improve health, but also open new markets for agricultural producers. Projections show rising trends in consumption of livestock, dairy, and other foods that make intensive use of energy and cereals, with worrisome implications for global food security and the environment. Thus it will also be important to work with consumer, public health, and environmental groups to find ways of encouraging people to adopt sustainable patterns of food consumption.

Create an Environment in Which Cooperation Can Thrive

• *Focus on partnerships among agriculture, nutrition, and health.* Professionals in agriculture, nutrition, and health speak different "languages," and efforts will be needed to overcome this barrier. These efforts will have to start at the time of professional training, through, for example, interdisciplinary problem-based learning approaches. National governments, farmers, healthcare workers, nutritionists, environmental groups, civil society organizations, educators, researchers, and the private sector all have important roles to play in leveraging agriculture for improved nutrition and health and should work together to achieve common goals. Special efforts should be made to ensure that the nutrition sector, which is often given short shrift, is an equal partner. Global and regional institutions that play important roles in the governance of the agriculture, nutrition, and health sectors may need to be reformed for greater effectiveness and integration of efforts.

• *Develop mutual accountability mechanisms among the three sectors.* It is important to promote openness and transparency and to develop clear guidelines for stakeholder responsibilities and resource allocation in agriculture, nutrition, and health. Leaders in the three sectors can create incentives that will make it easier for people in those sectors to work together.

• *Correct market failures.* Markets alone cannot achieve socially optimal agriculture, nutrition, and health outcomes. It is increasingly clear that agricultural and other policies have a range of benefits and costs for health, nutrition, and the environment that market prices do not reflect, especially given people's lack of information and knowledge. We need to do a better job of taking into account the true value—positive and negative—of nutritious foods, health services, and environmentally beneficial agricultural practices. Policymakers should use public policies— such as investments, subsidies, education, trade, and tax policies—to help correct these market failures and promote policy coherence at all levels.

- *Use communication and advocacy to bring about change.* Although there is wide interest in reducing undernutrition, converting goodwill into action can be difficult. Communication and advocacy can play an important role in increasing the visibility of nutrition issues, generating interest among agriculture and health professionals, stimulating action at all levels—global, regional, national, and local—and highlighting the important and interlinked roles played by all three sectors.

Recent food crises and protracted food inflation in many parts of the world have attracted renewed attention to agriculture. This is a useful moment to ask whether new ways of thinking and taking action can make agriculture more effective in promoting a more prosperous, healthy, and well-nourished world, while being mindful of its impact on the environment. This moment thus represents a window of opportunity for finding new solutions to longstanding problems of poor nutrition and health—solutions that could go a long way toward helping achieve all of the Millennium Development Goals and even surpassing them.

It is important to remember that agricultural growth alone will not eradicate undernutrition and ill health—specific interventions such as nutrition programs targeted at children under age two and improved healthcare services for underserved populations are still needed. Moreover, these kinds of safety net programs, as well as education and health services, infrastructure, trade policies, and other factors, make up the larger context within which advances in agriculture, nutrition, and health will take place. Changes in these factors will also make a difference to how well the linkages among agriculture, nutrition, and health operate.

In the coming decades, we are likely to face a more volatile world. Climate change, shifting diets, rising population, threats of water scarcity, and other factors will make leveraging agriculture for nutrition and health ever more challenging. We should anticipate these events and view them as opportunities to promote the structural changes needed to achieve a new balance, with more attention given to sustainable agriculture, improved health status, and better nutrition for all age groups.

Reference

FAO (Food and Agriculture Organization of the United Nations). 2010. *State of Food Insecurity in the World 2010.* Rome.

Contributors

Kwaw S. Andam (kandam@worldbank.org) is an economist at the World Bank, Washington, DC.

Felix A. Asante (fasante@isser.edu.gh) is a senior research fellow at the Institute of Statistical, Social and Economic Research, University of Ghana, Legon.

Kwadwo Asenso-Okyere (k.asenso-okyere@cgiar.org) is director of the Eastern and Southern Africa Regional Office of the International Food Policy Research Institute, Addis Ababa, Ethiopia.

Julia Behrman (j.behrman@cgiar.org) is a research analyst in the Poverty, Health, and Nutrition Division of the International Food Policy Research Institute, Washington, DC.

Todd Benson (t.benson@cgiar.org) is a senior research fellow in the Development Strategy and Governance Division of the International Food Policy Research Institute, Kampala, Uganda.

Howarth Bouis (h.bouis@cgiar.org) is the program director of HarvestPlus, Washington, DC.

Clemens Breisinger (c.breisinger@cgiar.org) is a research fellow in the Development Strategy and Governance Division of the International Food Policy Research Institute, Washington, DC.

Joanna Brzeska (j.brzeska@cgiar.org) is a consultant for the International Food Policy Research Institute, Washington, DC.

Catherine Chiang (c.chiang@cgiar.org) is a research analyst in the Environment and Production Technology Division of the International Food Policy Research Institute, Washington, DC.

Olivier Ecker (o.ecker@cgiar.org) is a postdoctoral fellow in the Development Strategy and Governance Division of the International Food Policy Research Institute, Washington, DC.

Shenggen Fan (s.fan@cgiar.org) is director general of the International Food Policy Research Institute, Washington, DC.

Heidi Fritschel (h.fritschel@cgiar.org) is an editor in the Communications Division of the International Food Policy Research Institute, Washington, DC.

Stuart Gillespie (s.gillespie@cgiar.org) is a senior research fellow in the Poverty, Health, and Nutrition Division of the International Food Policy Research Institute, based in Geneva, Switzerland.

Delia Grace (d.grace@cgiar.org) is a veterinary epidemiologist and food safety specialist at the International Livestock Research Institute, Nairobi, Kenya.

Corinna Hawkes (corinnahawkes@o2.co.uk) is a consultant on food and nutrition policy and a fellow at the Centre for Food Policy, City University London.

Derek Headey (d.headey@cgiar.org) is a research fellow in the Development Strategy and Governance Division of the International Food Policy Research Institute, based in Addis Ababa, Ethiopia.

John Hoddinott (j.hoddinott@cgiar.org) is deputy division director of the Poverty, Health, and Nutrition Division of the International Food Policy Research Institute, Washington, DC. He is also a senior research fellow.

Yassir Islam (y.islam@cgiar.org) is the communications head for HarvestPlus, Washington, DC.

Suneetha Kadiyala (s.kadiyala@cgiar.org) is a research fellow in the Poverty, Health, and Nutrition Division of the International Food Policy Research Institute, New Delhi, India.

Kenneth L. Leonard (kleonard@arec.umd.edu) is an associate professor in the Department of Agricultural and Resource Economics at the University of Maryland, College Park, United States.

John McDermott (j.mcdermott@cgiar.org) is director of the CGIAR Research Program on Agriculture for Improved Nutrition and Health led by the International Food Policy Research Institute, Washington, DC.

Paul E. McNamara (mcnamar1@illinois.edu) is an associate professor in the Department of Agricultural and Consumer Economics, the Department of Family Medicine, and the Division of Nutritional Sciences at the University of Illinois, Urbana-Champaign, United States.

Ruth Meinzen-Dick (r.meinzen-dick@cgiar.org) is a senior research fellow in the Environment and Production Technology Division of the International Food Policy Research Institute, Washington, DC.

Purnima Menon (p.menon@cgiar.org) is a research fellow in the Poverty, Health, and Nutrition Division of the International Food Policy Research Institute, New Delhi, India.

Siwa Msangi (s.msangi@cgiar.org) is a senior research fellow in the Environment and Production Technology Division of the International Food Policy Research Institute, Washington, DC.

Robert K. N. Mwadime (rmwadime@fhi360.org) is the senior regional nutrition advisor for the Food and Nutrition Technical Assistance II Project (FANTA-2), Kamapla, Uganda.

Clare Narrod (cnarrod@umd.edu) is a research scientist and risk analysis program manager at the Joint Institute for Food Safety and Applied Nutrition, University of Maryland, College Park, United States.

Robert Paarlberg (rpaarlberg@wellesley.edu) is the Betty Freyhof Johnson Class of 1944 Professor of Political Science at Wellesley College, Massachusetts, United States, and adjunct professor of public policy at the Harvard Kennedy School, Cambridge, Massachusetts.

Rajul Pandya-Lorch (r.pandya-lorch@cgiar.org) is head of the 2020 Vision Initiative and chief of staff in the Director General's Office of the International Food Policy Research Institute, Washington, DC.

Karl Pauw (k.pauw@cgiar.org) is a postdoctoral fellow in the Development Strategy and Governance Division of the International Food Policy Research Institute, based in Lilongwe, Malawi.

Per Pinstrup-Andersen (pp94@cornell.edu) is the H. E. Babcock Professor of Food, Nutrition, and Public Policy at Cornell University, Ithaca, New York, and a World Food Prize Laureate.

Agnes Quisumbing (a.quisumbing@cgiar.org) is a senior research fellow in the Poverty, Health, and Nutrition Division of the International Food Policy Research Institute, Washington, DC.

Mark W. Rosegrant (m.rosegrant@cgiar.org) is director of the Environment and Production Technology Division of the International Food Policy Research Institute (IFPRI) and interim director of the CGIAR Research Program on Policies, Institutions and Markets led by IFPRI, Washington, DC.

Devesh Roy (d.roy@cgiar.org) is a research fellow in the Markets, Trade, and Institutions Division of the International Food Policy Research Institute, Washington, DC.

Marie T. Ruel (m.ruel@cgiar.org) is director of the Poverty, Health, and Nutrition Division of the International Food Policy Research Institute, Washington, DC.

Brenda Shenute Namugumya (brendashenute@yahoo.co.uk) is a public nutrition specialist with the Regional Centre for Quality Health Care, attached to the Food and Nutrition Technical Assistance II Project (FANTA-2), Kampala, Uganda.

Jifar Tarekegn (jifar_t@yahoo.com) is a graduate student in the Department of Agricultural Economics, Texas A&M University, College Station, United States.

Paul Thangata (p.thangata@cgiar.org) is a research fellow in the Eastern and Southern Africa Regional Office of the International Food Policy Research Institute, Addis Ababa, Ethiopia.

James Thurlow (thurlow@wider.unu.edu) is a research fellow at the United Nations University World Institute for Development Economics Research, Helsinki, Finland. Previously, he was a research fellow in the Development Strategy and Governance Division of the International Food Policy Research Institute, Washington, DC.

Marites Tiongco (m.tiongco@cgiar.org) is a research fellow in the Markets, Trade, and Institutions Division of the International Food Policy Research Institute, Washington, DC.

Pippa Chenevix Trench (p.chenevixtrench@cgiar.org) previously served as a research fellow in the Markets, Trade, and Institutions Division of the International Food Policy Research Institute, Washington, DC.

John M. Ulimwengu (j.ulimwengu@cgiar.org) is a research fellow in the West and Central Africa Office of the International Food Policy Research Institute, Washington, DC.

Joachim von Braun (jvonbraun@uni-bonn.de) is director of the Center for Development Research and professor of economic and technological change at the University of Bonn, Germany.

Printed in Great Britain
by Amazon.co.uk, Ltd.,
Marston Gate.